Problems with Temperature Regulation during Exercise

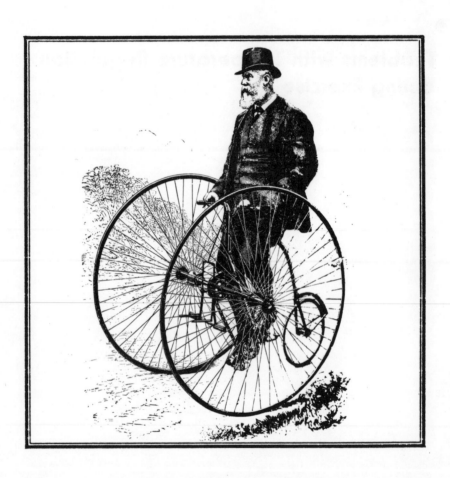

Viscount Bury

Problems with Temperature Regulation during Exercise

edited by

Ethan R. Nadel

John B. Pierce Foundation Laboratory
and
Yale University School of Medicine
New Haven, Connecticut

1977

ACADEMIC PRESS INC. New York San Francisco London
A Subsidiary of Harcourt Brace Jovanovich, Publishers

ACADEMIC PRESS RAPID MANUSCRIPT REPRODUCTION

ACADEMIC PRESS, INC.
111 Fifth Avenue, New York, New York 10003

United Kingdom Edition published by
ACADEMIC PRESS, INC. (LONDON) LTD.
24/28 Oval Road, London NW1

Library of Congress Cataloging in Publication Data

Main entry under title:

Problems with temperature regulation during exercise.

    Proceedings of a symposium held in conjunction
with the American College of Sports Medicine meeting,
Anaheim, Calif., May 1976.
    Includes indexes.
       1.   Exercise—Physiological aspects—Congresses.
2.   Body temperature—Regulation—Congresses.
I.   Nadel, Ethan R.   II.   American College of Sports
Medicine.
QP301.P76   612'.044   77-4301
ISBN 0–12–513550–5

PRINTED IN THE UNITED STATES OF AMERICA

CONTENTS

LIST OF CONTRIBUTORS

GEORGE L. BRENGELMANN Department of Physiology and Biophysics, University of Washington School of Medicine, Seattle, Washington

STEVEN M. HORVATH Institute of Environmental Stress, University of California, Santa Barbara, California

JOHN W. MITCHELL Department of Mechanical Engineering, University of Wisconsin, Madison, Wisconsin

ETHAN R. NADEL John B. Pierce Foundation Laboratory, and Departments of Epidemiology and Public Health and Physiology, Yale University School of Medicine, New Haven, Connecticut

MICHAEL R. ROBERTS John B. Pierce Foundation Laboratory, and Department of Epidemiology and Public Health, Yale University School of Medicine, New Haven, Connecticut

LORING B. ROWELL Department of Physiology and Biophysics, University of Washington School of Medicine, Seattle, Washington

JAN A. J. STOLWIJK John B. Pierce Foundation Laboratory, and Department of Epidemiology and Public Health, Yale University School of Medicine, New Haven, Connecticut

C. BRUCE WENGER John B. Pierce Foundation Laboratory, and Department of Epidemiology and Public Health, Yale University School of Medicine, New Haven, Connecticut

LIST OF CONTRIBUTORS

PREFACE

This volume of seven chapters considers various aspects of a specialized problem within the broader areas of temperature regulation and exercise physiology. These chapters represent summaries of the topics of a symposium entitled Problems of Temperature Regulation during Exercise, which was held in conjunction with the American College of Sports Medicine meeting in Anaheim, California, May 1976. The audience of this symposium, and the intended audience for this book, included students, teachers, physicians, and scientists interested in various aspects of exercise, thermal or circulatory physiology, the biophysics of heat transfer, and/or physiological control and regulation in general. Although the symposium concentrated on problems of human temperature regulation during exercise, many of the findings and much of the discussion could be applicable to any animal that regulates its internal body temperature, making allowances for differences in response capabilities across species.

The topics of the symposium, and of this book, were selected specifically to present a logical progression in the discussion of thermal control mechanisms and their activation during the stress of exercise. The participants were selected with this in mind, since they have consistently demonstrated their abilities to approach problems of physiological control and regulation in an analytical rather than a descriptive manner. With advancements in the techniques of measurement, it is understandable that there should have been a quantum step in productivity in the last decade or two. However, a quantum step in the level of knowledge does not necessarily follow. In order for the latter to occur, there must be new approaches to old problems. This is what has been demonstrated in the work of these individuals in their studies of different aspects of temperature regulation during exercise. Rather than considering physiological measurements on a temporal basis, they have generally placed physiological variables into their appropriate cause and effect loci within either mathematical or conceptual working models, thereby providing the basis upon which entirely new experiments were designed and carried out.

It should be pointed out that the contributors were conscripts rather than volunteers. Each was asked if he would participate and was assigned a topic within his area of expertise. Fortunately, each accepted the task willingly. Because of the rapid method of publishing, the material in each essay is up to date. This is a considerable advantage to both the authors, who are able to integrate recent information with older data, and to the reader, who is able to have a synopsis of current ideas in this field at his fingertips.

There are a number of people who aided in the preparation of this collection of essays and who deserve special recognition. The participants of the symposium, besides providing current material, were most helpful in providing lucid, descriptive, and analytical manuscripts. Frances Ahern, Jerleen Forbes, and Gertrude Vickstrom were invaluable in the laying out and typing of the book. Wayne Chappell did much of the drafting and photography work and Nancy Bavor found the Daumier prints in the bowels of the Yale Medical Library, which generously allowed us to reproduce them. Some of the ideas and research that appear were made possible by NIH Grants ES-00123, and National Academy of Sciences Marsh Fund Award. The American College of Sports Medicine sponsored the symposium (i.e., put it on the program and provided the participants with their expenses); this volume would never have been possible without their support. Finally, I extend special thanks to the staffs of the John B. Pierce Foundation Laboratory and the Departement de Physiologie Humaine for time, space, and advice.

A Brief Overview...

Ethan R. Nadel

The consideration of a specific problem area within the relatively broad field of temperature regulation may seem to be
overly specialized to warrant discussion as a separate entity.
In fact, this particular consideration arrives at the heart of
the study of thermoregulatory mechanisms in humans. Exercise represents the single condition that provides a maximal
strain to most regulatory systems under normal circumstances.
A reliable technique toward understanding any control system
is providing that system with a load and observing the quality
and quantity of adjustor action. During exposure to extreme
environments the body is rarely faced with thermal loads in
excess of 200 W. Furthermore, the body is usually protected
from environmental exposures this severe by its ability to
make behavioral adjustments (such as changing the insulative
layer of clothing or escaping from the noxious environment) in
response to the early sensation of extreme conditions. In
contrast, thermal loads that are imposed upon an average individual during exercise, as a result of the production of heat
in the contracting muscles, can be in excess of 600-800 watts
for extended periods and in excess of 1000 watts for limited
periods. In the first instance, distribution of this heat
throughout the body is sufficient to raise the body core temperature of an average-sized individual by 1.0° C every five
to eight minutes if no thermoregulatory responses were
activated. Increases in internal body temperature of more
than 3.0° C can be accompanied by central nervous system
dysfunction, circulatory failure and, eventually, irreversible
tissue damage and death. Thus, without the activation of
thermoregulatory mechanisms, moderate exercise in humans
would be limited to fifteen minutes or less. However, it is
well established that specialized areas in the brain sense the
increased body temperatures and activate appropriate efferent

responses which counteract excessive hyperthermia. Because of the integrated thermoregulatory response, moderate exercise can be sustained for extended periods, with the internal body temperature reaching a new steady state rather than continuing to climb. In this case the heat produced during exercise is balanced by the heat dissipated to the environment.

The questions of which temperatures are the ones that are monitored by the body and whether it is heat flow that is regulated rather than temperature and whether there are important non-thermal stimuli which contribute to the integrated thermoregulatory response during exercise and whether the latter problem constitutes a shift in the "set-point" during exercise are questions that are referred to indirectly rather than directly in the following chapters. Although these questions may be considered as "fringe" rather than central to the overall discussion of temperature regulation in humans, they are important enough to receive some attention, and I shall do so briefly in the following paragraphs.

It is well established that there are specialized nervous structures which are responsive to temperature and/or to temperature change. Temperature sensitive free nerve endings have been found in abundance near the skin surface (4) and in the preoptic area of the hypothalamus (8). Because of the characteristics of these neurons and the abundant information that discrete changes of skin or hypothalamic temperature elicit appropriate thermal defense reactions, the skin and hypothalamus have been generally accepted as the primary areas of sensation and subsequent transmission of thermal information to the thermoregulatory center, which is also assigned to the hypothalamus. It should be pointed out that in certain animals temperature regulatory responses have also been identified with changes in the spinal cord temperature (11). Although spinal thermosensitivity may be important in the integrated thermoregulatory activity of these animals, it is not known whether the spinal cord in humans has any role other than that of a relay station.

Measurement of hypothalamic temperature is, of course, not possible in humans. This has resulted in different techniques for estimation of hypothalamic temperature in

experimental conditions. Since the hypothalamic temperature
is mostly determined by the temperature of arterial blood
(since rates of hypothalamic heat production and hypothalamic
blood flow are relatively constant), it follows that arterial (or
even central venous) blood temperature should provide a good
approximation of hypothalamic temperature. Simultaneous
measurements on animals bear this out (3). However, it is
usually not practical to monitor central blood temperature in
humans during exercise. The most reliable "non-invasive"
estimate of central blood temperature in humans is esophageal
temperature. The site of measurement is near the heart and
great vessels, adjacent to the left atrium. Since there is not
a great amount of insulative tissue in this area, there is a
relatively low inertia and a rapid response to a change in
thermal load. Esophageal temperature is independent of ambient or facial temperature, whereas the tympanic membrane
temperature is not (6). Rectal temperature, also often used
as an approximation of brain temperature, has the disadvantage of being slow to respond to a change in thermal load.
Thus, for studies during a thermal transient, rectal temperature is a poor indicator of brain temperature. For the past
twenty years, physiologists have known that the temperature
in the esophagus is a relatively close reflection of central
arterial blood temperature. It is curious that few studies involving temperature regulation in humans have taken advantage of this fortuitous relationship.

In humans, indirect physiological evidence shows that the
thermal sensors on the skin are not distributed evenly over
the surface, but tend to be more concentrated than predicted
according to surface area on the face and less concentrated
than predicted on the lower arms and lower legs. This is true
for both cold (2) and warmth perception (7). Thus, when measuring the average temperature of the skin it is important to
consider both area and sensitivity weighting in the computation. The most accurate factors for weighting local skin
temperatures in the computation of $\bar{T}_{sk}$ are as follows:

$$\bar{T}_{sk} = 0.21\ T_{face} + 0.17\ T_{abdomen} + 0.11\ T_{chest} +$$
$$0.10\ T_{back} + 0.15\ T_{thigh} + 0.08\ T_{calf} +$$
$$0.12\ T_{upper\ arm} + 0.06\ T_{lower\ arm}$$

Since the physiological response to a change in load is related to the magnitude of the physiological (rather than the environmental) change, an optimal evaluation of the physiological control of the heat loss response in humans should consider the relation between the body temperatures (the important afferent information to the central nervous system integrator in the hypothalamus) and the skin blood flow or sweating rate. Thus, sweating and skin blood flow data are usefully plotted against internal temperature rather than time or exercise intensity, which are not the primary stimuli. This allows the visualization of the control system as a control system, where stimulus produces response; the conceptual model has both predictive and physiological validity. From such a depiction, one can make further determinations about the system, such as how it is modified in different conditions. For instance, a question that has not been satisfactorily answered to this time is whether the decrease in sweating in a prolonged exposure to heat or exercise is the result of a change in the central nervous system "set" or threshold temperature for sweating or whether the decrease is the result of a decrease in sweat gland responsiveness to a given neuroglandular signal. By evaluating the stimulus-response characteristics in different conditions rather than the temporal pattern of response, it would be obvious which of the above possibilities provides the better explanation. This concept of characterizing thermoregulatory responses is discussed and illustrated in greater detail in chapters 3 and 5.

It is important to make the differentiation between the hyperthermia of exercise and fever. The increased body core temperature during exercise constitutes an offset from the idealized, regulated core temperature. This elevated temperature triggers a heat dissipation response which is related to the magnitude of the offset (this concept will be discussed in detail in Chapter 3). The important point here is that the regulated internal body temperature is the same during exercise as it is during rest. In his classic paper of 1938, Marius Nielsen observed that the elevation of internal body temperature during exercise was proportional to the intensity of exercise in any individual (9). He and others assumed that the new steady state core temperature

was a regulated one, and for years it was generally agreed
that exercise was accompanied by an elevated "set-point". .
Sid Robinson (10), in 1949, clarified this point somewhat by
demonstrating the proportional relationship between sweating
rate and rectal temperature, when skin temperature was constant. These data allowed the interpretation that sweating
rate was a controlled variable, with the internal temperature
acting as the primary feedback element. This latter explanation does not require a shift in the "set-point" or regulated
temperature, but rather provides for an internal temperature
which is regulated about a constant set temperature, with increases in sweating rate at higher body temperatures serving
to attempt to re-establish this regulated temperature. In the
steady state of exercise, when the rate of heat production is
high, the core temperature is driven to the point where it
stimulates the sweating response. Increased sweating results
in increased heat dissipation via evaporation, ultimately
balancing the heat production. When the heat production is
balanced by the heat dissipation, there is no longer any
change in the body's storage of heat and internal body temperature remains constant.

Fever, on the other hand, is generally thought to be the
consequence of an elevation in the regulated internal body
temperature. This was recognized about 100 years ago by
Liebermeister (5), who stated that the body thermostat was
re-set to a higher level in fever. Thus, in the presence of
certain pathological conditions, the body makes regulatory
adjustments in order to maintain its core temperature at an
elevated (above normal) level. The most convincing data
that I have seen in verification of this assumption were
published recently by Stitt et al. using a rabbit model (13).
In a cool environment a single injection of prostaglandin E_1
into the animal's hypothalamus caused the animal to increase
its rate of heat production, driving the internal (rectal and
hypothalamic) body temperatures up by around $1.0^{\circ}C$.
Figure 1 describes the metabolic rate as a function of hypothalamic temperature, illustrating the shift in metabolic rate
toward higher temperatures following intrahypothalamic injection of the prostaglandin. The magnitude of the shift is
shown at the point of zero metabolism, and amounts to somewhat more than $1.0^{\circ}C$ of hypothalamic temperature, thereby

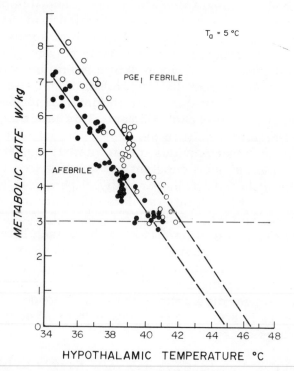

FIG. 1. Change in metabolic rate with respect
to hypothalamic temperature in afebrile and
febrile rabbits. Note that while thermosensitivity is similar, the response threshold (and set
temperature at zero metabolic rate) has
increased in febrile animals. Modified from
Stitt, et al. (13).

accounting for the entire febrile response in these conditions.
This can be considered as an upward shift in the regulated
temperature or the "set-point". Recent observations in our
laboratory have verified this concept for humans during
exercise. Figure 2 illustrates an upward shift in the internal
temperature threshold for vasodilation on a day when the
subject complained of "sore throat and general feeling of
malaise". The blood flow data revealed that this subject was
running a sub-clinical fever of about 0.5° C. This does not
imply an additional elevation superimposed upon the core temperature increase during exercise, but rather a greater latency
in heat dissipation response with increased core temperature.

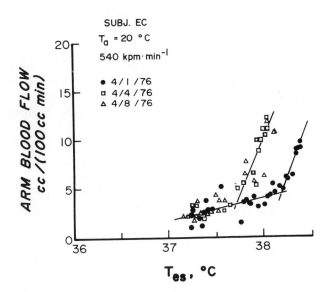

*FIG. 2. Change in forearm blood flow with
respect to esophageal temperature in a subject
during leg exercise in normal (open symbols)
and febrile (filled symbols) conditions.*

   Now and then the question arises of whether the body
regulates its heat content or heat flow rather than its internal
temperature. In fact, many an otherwise-knowledgeable
scientist will incorrectly describe homeothermy as the process of "heat regulation". Since temperature and heat content are proportional when the mass and specific heat of the
body are constant, it would appear that heat regulation is an
adequate description of the maintenance of the constancy of
internal body temperature. However, this description fails
as one makes a closer examination of experimental data.

The most damaging evidence against a heat regulation theory comes from the ever-increasing number of studies investigating the sensitivity of the controller. This type of study involves the heating or cooling of a small mass of tissue in the preoptic area of the anterior hypothalamus by perfusing an implanted thermode with water of a known temperature. The animal's regulatory response to small displacements of hypothalamic temperature can be so great as to drive deep body temperature more than 1.0° C in the opposite direction within 15 minutes (12). This type of response is only possible if the heated or cooled tissue is highly sensitive to its own temperature and if the temperature within this tissue is the body's regulated temperature. The response to a relatively small displacement of hypothalamic temperature results in a heat flow from the body which is far in excess of the heat flow into the body. If heat content or heat flow were the regulated variable, this imbalance could not occur.

The heat flow vs. temperature controversy has hopefully been settled by the recent arguments of Cabanac (1). He pointed out that body mass varies greatly both between species and in a single individual during growth. If body heat content were regulated, for instance, the body temperature should be inversely related to the mass during development or after sudden changes in mass (following a diet, for instance). Of course, this is not the case. The body has no known sensors of heat content per se, or even of heat flow. At any stage during growth and development, body temperature is tightly regulated and is independent of mass. Further, body temperature is independent of the mass which receives the circulation...i.e., the body mass receiving blood flow in a warm environment is considerably greater than that in a cold environment, when blood flow to peripheral tissues is minimal. In the latter case the heat content of the body (mean body temperature times the mass times the specific heat) can be less than 90 per cent of that in a vasodilated individual.

In fairness to proponents of a heat flow regulation theory, it is conceivable that the body has the capability of assessing heat flow by sensing the temperature gradient across a given field. Since mass and thermal conductivity are constant, the temperature differential would provide the heat flow. This is a similar system of measurement to that employed by commercially available heat flow discs, where the temperature gradient across a known mass yields the heat flow. If this were the case, for the body to accurately and continuously monitor heat flow, it should have thermal sensors at different depths in the epidermal layer. Further, it should be able to integrate thermal information as well as to take account of the depth of the sensors which are supplying the information. Although plausible, this description requires a complex feedback and integration network and substitutes for a rather simple network which monitors temperature solely. The heat flow regulation theory also does not account for the findings of the thermode studies. Therefore, until a more convincing argument is set forth, we are bound by the classical view that temperature is the regulated variable rather than heat content or heat flow.

Specifically and briefly stated, the problem that this book is concerned with is the means and ways the body has to dissipate the tremendous thermal load generated during exercise, thereby preventing it from burning up from the inside.

In the following chapters the physical means by which heat is transferred both within the body and between the body and its environment are described, and the physiological systems which control the rates of transfer are discussed. Also discussed are conditions in which the controlling systems are limited in their abilities to transfer heat and conditions in which the controlling systems adapt in their capabilities. Although this volume is broad in its scope, there are certain deficits, most of which are the consequence of deficits in our knowledge of the interaction between control systems. Some of these deficits, some points of disagreement and some unanswered questions will be expanded in the final chapter.

References

1. Cabanac, M. Temperature regulation. Ann. Rev. Physiol. 37: 415-439, 1975.
2. Crawshaw, L. I., E. R. Nadel, J. A. J. Stolwijk and B. A. Stamford. Effect of local cooling on sweating rate and cold sensation. Pflugers Archiv. 354: 19-27, 1975.
3. Hayward, J. N. and M. A. Baker. Role of cerebral arterial blood in the regulation of brain temperature in the monkey. Am. J. Physiol. 215: 389-403, 1968.
4. Hensel, H., A. Iggo and I. Witt. A quantitative study of sensitive cutaneous thermoreceptors with C afferent fibers. J. Physiol. (London) 153: 113-126, 1960.
5. Liebermeister, C. von. Handbuch der Pathologie und Therapie des Fiebers. Leipzig, Vogel, 1875.
6. Nadel, E. R. and S. M. Horvath. Comparison of tympanic membrane and deep body temperatures in man. Life Sci. 9: 869-875, 1970.
7. Nadel, E. R., J. W. Mitchell and J. A. J. Stolwijk. Differential thermal sensitivity in the human skin. Pflugers Archiv. 340: 71-76, 1973.
8. Nakayama, T., H. T. Hammel, J. D. Hardy and J. S. Eisenman. Thermal stimulation and electrical activity of single units of the preoptic region. Am. J. Physiol. 204: 1122-1126, 1963.
9. Nielsen, M. Die Regulation der Korpertemperatur bei Muskelarbeit. Skand. Arch. Physiol. 79: 193-230, 1938.
10. Robinson, S. Physiological adjustments to heat. In: Physiology of Heat Regulation and the Science of Clothing. C. H. Newburg (Ed), W. B. Saunders Co, Philadelphia, 1949, 193-231.
11. Simon, E., W. Rautenberg, R. Thauer and M. Iriki. Die Auslosung von Kaltezittern durch lokale Kuhlung im Wirbelkanal. Pflugers Archiv. 381: 309-331, 1963.
12. Stitt, J. T. and J. D. Hardy. Thermoregulation in the squirrel monkey (Saimiri Sciureus). J. Appl. Physiol. 31: 48-54, 1971.
13. Stitt, J. T., J. D. Hardy and J. A. J. Stolwijk. PGE_1 fever: its effect on thermoregulation at different low ambient temperatures. Am. J. Physiol. 227: 622-629, 1974.

Energy Exchanges During Exercise

John W. Mitchell

Introduction

The response of the human system to exercise can be visualized as a chain reaction originating at the working muscle and ultimately involving the cardiovascular, respiratory, and thermoregulatory systems. The driving force is the demand to produce mechanical work via the oxidation of nutrients. Fuel and oxygen supplies are available as stores in the muscle tissue for short term exercise, while for longer periods these supplies must be transported to the muscle by the blood stream. The muscle blood flow increases to meet the oxygen demand of the working muscle, and the oxygen extraction per unit volume of blood increases. This conversion of fuel energy produces heat in addition to mechanical work and the heat in part goes to increase the local tissue temperatures, is transferred to the blood stream, and is conducted to the surrounding tissue. The temperature of the muscle is a result of a balance between these thermal energy flows.

The increased oxygen uptake by the muscle reduces the oxygen content of the venous blood. In the lungs, increased ventilation is required to replace the oxygen consumed and saturate the arterial blood. Work is required by the chest muscles to provide this increased ventilation. In addition, the increased air flow transfers some of the thermal energy produced at the muscle from the body by both convection and evaporation in the respiratory passage.

The thermal state of the body as a result of exercise is one of generally elevated temperatures. Working muscle temperatures are quite higher than in the resting state. The temperature of the venous blood is increased by heat transfer and consequently arterial blood and core temperatures are raised. The blood flow transports thermal energy to the skin, where it is transferred to the environment by convection, radiation and evaporation.

All of these adjustments are interrelated, and together constitute the homeokinetic response to exercise. It is the objective of this paper to describe a) the physical mechanisms of thermal energy production at the working muscle, and b) the transfers of this thermal energy to the environment.

Basic Relations For Working Muscle

In this section, the relationships governing the oxygen and energy demands of working muscle will be developed following Mitchell, et al (6). These relations will be used to indicate the partitioning of the various oxygen and energy forms from the muscle.

The oxygen utilization in the working muscle is shown schematically in Figure 1. Oxygen is carried into the muscle

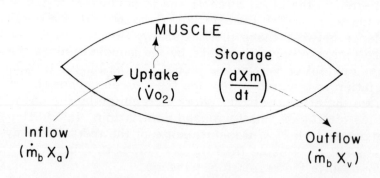

FIG. 1.   *Schematic of oxygen flows for working muscle.*

capillary bed by the arterial blood flow. Oxygen uptake occurs
through aerobic metabolic processes in the muscle, and the
oxygen content of the venous blood is diminished. During
transients of exercise, oxygen may be released from the muscle myoglobin stores. The relation between these terms is
given by the conservation of matter principle applied to the
oxygen in a unit mass of muscle which states that

$$Rate\ of\ change\ of\ storage \atop of\ oxygen = Inflow \atop of\ oxygen - Outflow \atop of\ oxygen$$

or

$$\frac{dx_m}{dt} = \dot{m}_b (x_a - x_v) - \dot{V}_{0_2, m} \qquad (Eq\ 1)$$

where x_m is the oxygen stored in the muscle myoglobin, $\dot{m}_b$ is
the muscle blood flow, x_a and x_v are the arterial and venous
oxygen concentration in the blood flowing through the muscle,
$\dot{V}_{0_2, m}$ is the rate of oxygen uptake by the muscle.

The release of oxygen stored in the myoglobin and hemo-
globins contributes to oxygen deficit observed at the onset of
exercise. However, these stores are small, and can contribute about 0.5 liters of oxygen at most. Increased oxygen
uptake results from the combination of increased muscle blood
flow and increased extraction (arterio-venous difference). The
major effect is the increase in blood flow, which can rise by
a factor of 20 to 30, in contrast to extraction, which can increase by a factor of four at most.

The energy flows for the working muscle are shown schematically in Figure 2. In addition to the oxygen supplied for
aerobic metabolism, there are releases of chemical energy
stores from the muscle. The metabolic processes convert
chemical energy into mechanical work and thermal energy.
During the onset, thermal energy is stored in the muscle mass,
thereby raising the muscle temperature. Heat is transferred
from the hotter muscle to the surrounding tissue. The blood
enters the muscle at body (core) temperature, thermally
equilibrates with the muscle in the capillaries, and leaves
at muscle temperature. The relation between these terms is
the conservation of energy principle applied to the muscle

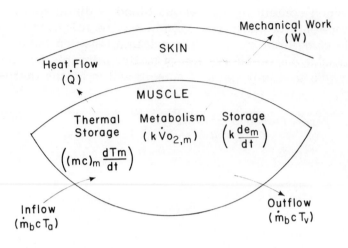

FIG. 2.   Schematic of energy flows for working muscle.

mass, which states

$$\text{Rate of change of storage of energy} = \text{Inflow of energy} - \text{Outflow of energy}$$

or

$$k\frac{de_m}{dt} + (mc)_m\frac{dT_m}{dt} = \dot{m}_b c(T_c - T_m) + k\dot{V}_{O_2,m} - W - Q$$

(Eq 2)

where e_m is the oxygen equivalent of the chemical energy stored in the muscle, k is a constant relating the conversion of oxygen to heat and work, $(mc)_m$ is the mass – specific heat product of the muscle, T_m and T_c are muscle and arterial (core) temperatures, c is the specific heat of the blood, W is the rate of mechanical work leaving the muscle, and Q is the rate of heat flow.

The release of phosphagen stores and the anaerobic gly-
colytic potential are the major contributors to the oxygen deficit, and can amount to 4 to 5 liters of oxygen. The major
path for the transfer of thermal energy from the working muscle
is through the increased blood flow.

The two relations can be combined to eliminate the muscle
oxygen consumption. The resulting relation may be used to
yield insight into the magnitude of the various terms:

$$k[\dot{m}_b(x_a - x_r) - \frac{de_m}{dt} - \frac{dx_m}{dt}] = W + Q + \dot{m}_b c(T_m - T_c) - (mc)_m \frac{dT_m}{dt}$$

$$(Eq\ 3)$$

The terms on the left side of Eq. 3 represent the oxygen
supplied to the muscle by the blood oxygen and chemical
stores. The stores are significant only during onset of exercise, and are used up in the first few minutes of exercise.
As a consequence, a cardiovascular steady state is achieved
rapidly. In contrast, the thermal response is considerably
slower. Thermal energy is stored not only in the muscle
mass, but in the rest of the body by the flow of the warmed
blood. It takes 20 to 30 minutes to achieve a steady thermal
state.

The oxygen consumption in the working muscle may rise to
3 to 4 l/min during heavy work, while the consumption in the
remaining portions of the body is 0.2 to 0.3 l/min. Thus,
the total oxygen uptake is essentially that of the working
muscle. The efficiency of conversion of this chemical energy
to mechanical work is defined as

$$\eta_m = W/\dot{V}_{O_2} \qquad (Eq\ 4)$$

The efficiency η_m is about 20 percent under optimal conditions such as on a cycle ergometer. For exercise such as
running or bicycling (3) and most sports the mechanical work
production, and thus the efficiency, is essentially zero. Thus,
from Eq. 3, it is seen that at least 80 percent of the energy
released by oxygen consumption must go to thermal forms and
ultimately, under steady conditions, be dissipated as heat
from the skin and respiratory tract.

These relationships are shown graphically for a typical exercise level in Fig. 3. The results are based on verified models for oxygen uptake and thermoregulation (6, 10), and are for the simulation of bicycle exercise. The top portion of Fig. 3 shows the cardiac response in comparison to the metabolic demand. The ventilation and oxygen consumption responses parallel the cardiac output. The deficit is quickly incurred, and the responses are relatively fast, with steady state reached in about 5 minutes.

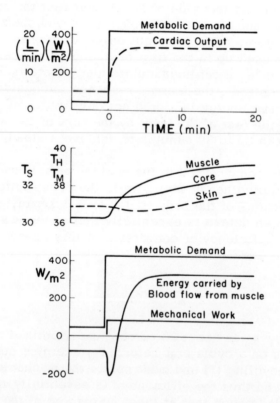

FIG. 3. *Response to onset of exercise.*

The temperature changes of muscle, skin and body core with exercise are shown in the center of Fig. 3.

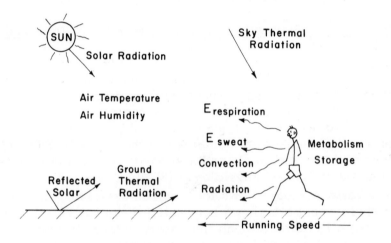

FIG. 4. *Energy flows for a person exercising in the outdoor environment.*

Leg muscle temperature (T_m) is initially lower than core temperature (T_H). The muscle temperature rises quite rapidly at the onset of exercise. The core temperature rises more slowly, and reflects the large amount of energy storage in the entire body mass. Skin temperature initially drops slightly due to increased convection resulting from the motion of the subject, and then gradually rises.

These temperature responses reach steady state in about 30 minutes.

The thermal energy transport via the blood flow is shown at the bottom of Fig. 3 in comparison with the metabolic demands and the mechanical work. The major portion of the energy produced by metabolic processes is carried away by the blood and distributed throughout the body. As discussed earlier, 20 percent of the energy at most leaves as mechanical work. A very small portion of the thermal energy produced is transported directly to the skin by conduction. Skin blood flow plays a major role in the distribution of the thermal energy.

Energy Transfer Between The Skin And Respiratory Tract And The Environment

In this section, the mechanisms of energy transfer from the lungs and skin to the environment will be discussed. The basic relations will first be presented, and then discussed in the context of energy flows for an exercising subject. More complete works on this subject are contained in the books by Fanger (3) and Åstrand and Rodahl (1) and a summary of the relations is in the Journal of Applied Physiology, (8).

The various energy flows for a person exercising in an outdoor environment are shown schematically in Fig. 4. These flows are all related through the energy balance principle, which states that the change in thermal energy storage equals the thermal energy generated by metabolism (M) plus the solar energy absorbed (So) and minus the outputs by mechanical work (W), the respiratory tract (E_{res}), convection (C), radiation (R), and the evaporation of sweat (E_{sw}). This equation is written as

$$(mc) \; \frac{dT_b}{dt} = M + So - W - E_{res} - C - R - E_{sw} \qquad (Eq \; 5)$$

where (mc) is the mass specific heat product of the person and T_b is mean body temperature.

The thermal inputs are metabolism and solar energy. The energy production by metabolism has been described earlier. For a person exercising outdoors, incident solar energy is absorbed at the skin surface, and is given by

$$So = \alpha \, A_p \, I \qquad (Eq \; 6)$$

where a is the solar absorptivity of the exposed skin, A_p the projected area, and I the incident solar insolation. The absorptivity of human skin is about 0.6. The projected area is the body area normal to the sun's rays, and ranges from about 0.3 m^2 for the sun overhead to 0.6 m^2 for the sun on the horizon. The solar insolation depends on time of day, season, and locality. For clear skies a value of 1000 W/m^2 is typical. Thus, solar heating can be significant for an exercising subject.

The energy loss from the respiratory tract occurs via two modes. There is an evaporative cooling effect as the relatively dry inspired air is humidified by evaporation of water from the respiration surfaces. In addition, there is convective cooling of the respiration tract as the inspired air is warmed. These losses depend on the levels of the inspired air temperature and humidity, and on the magnitude of the ventilation flow rate. The respiration loss is given by Fanger (3) and Mitchell et al. (5), as follows:

$$E_{res} = \dot{V}_e \ \rho [\lambda (\gamma_x - \gamma_a) + c_p (Te_x - T_a)] \qquad (Eq \ 7)$$

where V_e is the ventilatory flow rate, ρ and c_p the inspired air density and specific heat, λ the heat of vaporization of water, γ_{ex} and γ_a are the expired and ambient air absolute humidities, and T_{ex} and T_a the expired and ambient air temperatures.

The ventilation flow rate during exercise is proportional to oxygen consumption which is proportional to metabolism. Below about 75 percent of maximum oxygen consumption, the relation is given by Åstrand and Rodahl (1):

$$\dot{V}_e = 23 \ \dot{V}_{0_2} \qquad (Eq \ 8)$$

For exercising subjects over a wide range of ambient conditions, the expired air temperature has been found to remain essentially constant at 35°C. The humidity of the expired air has been found to depend on the humidity of the inspired air. An empirical relation that adequately describes this humidity change in the respiration tract is from McCutchan and Taylor (4):

$$\gamma_{ex} - \gamma_a = 0.029 - 0.8 \ \gamma_a \qquad in \ kg/kg \ air$$
$$(Eq \ 9)$$

The absolute humidity of the air can also be represented by its vapor pressure, Pa (mm Hg). These relations can be incorporated into Eq. 9, and the respiratory loss written as

$$E_{res} = 0.0023 \; M[(44-P_a) + 0.61 \; (35-T_a)] \qquad (Eq \; 10)$$

Convection is the transfer of heat from the skin surface to the surrounding air, with the heated fluid moved away by the motion. The expression for convection heat transfer is

$$C = h_c \; A_D (\bar{T}_s - T_a) \qquad (Eq \; 11)$$

where h_c is the convection coefficient and A_D the exposed skin area (the DuBois skin area). The heat transfer coefficient is a function of the relative motion between the subject and the ambient air. Nishi and Gagge (7) have evaluated both local and total body heat transfer coefficients for humans exercising on treadmills and bicycle ergometers and for free walking exercise. For free walking exercise up to 2 m/s, the heat transfer coefficient is given by

$$h_c = 8.6 \; V^{0.531} \qquad (Eq \; 12)$$

where h_c is measured in W/m^2 - C and V in m/s. Equation 12 indicates that the convection coefficient doubles for about a four-fold increase in running speed. The experiments on which Eq. 12 is based on are below 2 m/s, but convective heat transfer theory indicates that the relation would be reasonably accurate at higher velocities.

Radiation heat transfer is the net energy exchange between a surface and its surroundings through long wave electromagnetic emissions. Each surface emits energy proportional to the fourth power of its absolute temperature. The net exchange between a person and his surroundings is given by

$$R = \epsilon \; A_D F \sigma (\bar{T}_s^4 - T_r^4) \qquad (Eq \; 13)$$

where ϵ is the long wave (thermal) emissivity of the skin, F the view factor between the skin and the surroundings, σ the Stefan-Boltzmann constant (5.67×10^{-8} W/m^2-K^4), and $\bar{T}_s$ and T_r the absolute temperatures of the skin and surroundings. A perfect emitter has a long wave emissivity of unity and human skin is close to this with a value between 0.95 and 0.98. The view factor is a geometric factor that reflects the amount of energy emitted by the skin going directly to the surroundings. Shape factors for humans have been estimated at between 0.7 for sitting subjects and 0.85 for spread-eagle subjects (3). Radiant exchange is not usually the major heat loss term, and so extreme accuracy in the value for the view factor is not necessary. The radiant temperature of the surroundings is taken as the ambient air temperature under normal conditions.

Equation 13 can be expressed in a form similar to Eq. 11 for ease in calculation of heat loss. The radiation coefficient h_r is defined as

$$h_r = 4 \, \varepsilon \, F\sigma [(T_s + T_a)/2]^3 \qquad (Eq \ 14)$$

and thus

$$R = h_r \, A_D (\bar{T}_s - T_a) \qquad (Eq \ 15)$$

For moderate temperatures, Eq. 15 closely approximates Eq. 12. The form of Eq. 14 allows C and R to be added together as

$$C + R = (h_c + h_r) \, A_D \, (\bar{T}_s - T_a)$$

Evaporation of sweat from the surface of the skin is a major avenue of heat loss for an exercising subject. Sweat secretion is governed by the thermoregulatory system, and produced in response to skin and core temperature changes. The evaporation of sweat from the surface is governed by mechanisms similar to the convection of heat. The expression for convective evaporation is

$$E_{sw} = h_s \, A_w \, \lambda \, (\rho_s - \rho_a) \qquad (Eq \ 16)$$

where h_d is a diffusion coefficient related directly to the convection coefficient h_c, A_w is the wetted skin area, λ is the heat of vaporization of sweat, and ρ_s and ρ_a are the densities of the water vapor at the skin surface and ambient air, respectively. The wetted skin area is usually considerably less than the total skin area under most exercising conditions.

Equation 16 is usually rewritten to introduce the vapor pressure and combine some of the physical constants. In addition, the analogy relation between the diffusion and convection coefficients is employed to bring in the convection coefficient directly. Equation 16 can be rewritten as

$$E_{sw} = 2.2\, h_c\, A_w (P_s - P_a) \qquad (Eq\ 17)$$

where P_s and P_a are the vapor pressures in mm Hg, and h_c is the convection coefficient in $W/m^2 \cdot {}^\circ C$.

The role of these different mechanisms in the overall energy balance of an exercising subject can be best shown by example. The contribution of the various terms to the production and dissipation of heat will be computed for an exercising runner. It will be assumed that he is exercising steadily at 70% of his maximum output with an oxygen consumption of 2.8 l/min. This level approximates a pace of 8 minutes per mile, or a speed of 3.3 m/s (2). His core temperature would rise from a normal value of 37°C to about 37.9°C. The rise is essentially independent of the environmental temperature (9).

The runner will be assumed to be exercising wearing only shorts and in the sun. The entire metabolic energy generated by his exercise, 980 W, must be dissipated as heat since he does not do any external work. The solar energy absorbed by his bare skin surface is taken to be 140 W. The thermal results will be presented for different ambient air temperatures ranging from 10°C to 35°C and at 60% relative humidity.

The average skin temperature of the runner over this ambient temperature range is shown at the top of Fig. 5. It is seen that the mean skin temperature changes only 8°C over a 25°C change in ambient temperature. The variation of skin temperature with ambient temperature is essentially independent of the level of exercise (9). This is in contrast to the core temperature rise, which is essentially independent of the ambient conditions.

The partitioning of the energy generation and dissipation is shown at the bottom of Fig. 5. Under steady exercise, the sum of the energy transfers by respiration, radiation,

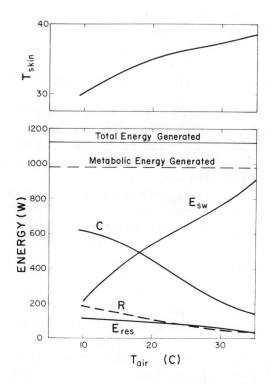

FIG. 5. *Partition of heat loss from an exercising person.*

convection, and sweating equals the production by metabolism and the absorption of solar energy. At the lowest ambient temperature (10°C), convection is the major mode of heat loss, and accounts for over 50% of the total. Radiation transfer and evaporation of sweat each comprise about 20% of the total loss, and the respiration loss is about 10%. The sweat loss at these low temperatures is relatively small. The difference in temperature between the skin and the ambient is relatively high, and thus the potential for heat loss by convection and radiation is high. The respiration loss is also relatively high due to the low absolute humidity of the inspired air.

At higher ambient temperatures, evaporation of sweat becomes a more important mode of heat loss. Skin temperatures rise with ambient temperature but cannot exceed core temperature. Thus, the potential for heat loss by convection, radiation, and sensible respiration decreases even though the heat transfer coefficients and the ventilation flow rate remain the same. Also, the absolute humidity (vapor pressure) of the ambient increases with temperature for a constant relative humidity, and thus the latent respiration loss decreases. At 35°C, 85% of the loss is by sweating and 90% of the total skin area is wet. This corresponds to a water loss of about 1.3 kg/hr.

The partitioning of these energy losses depends on the environmental variables other than temperature, but to a lesser degree. If the runner is shaded by clouds, 140 W less energy needs to be dissipated. At 30°C this corresponds to a 15% drop in required sweating rate.

Ambient humidity affects both the respiratory and evaporative heat loss. At an ambient of 30°C, if the relative humidity were 80%, the respiratory loss would drop by 25% from its value at 60% RH, while at 20% RH it would increase 60%. However, since radiation and convection losses are not affected, these changes would require corresponding changes in sweat loss to maintain thermal equilibrium. Thus the total water loss would remain the same. There would, however, be changes in the amount of skin area that is wet. At 60% RH and 30°C, 40% of the skin area is wet. At 80% RH, the skin wettedness would rise to 55%, while at 20% RH it would drop to 25%. Thus, different ambient humidities require different amounts of wetted skin to achieve the same evaporative loss, but only the comfort level is affected. Even at 100% RH, the skin wettedness would be only 75%, and thus the runner could exercise in this environment and dissipate heat.

Large changes in wind speed would produce relatively small changes in the partitioning of the energy loss. For example, a 10 mph head wind at 30°C would increase the convection coefficient and the corresponding convective heat loss by about 50%. However, the evaporative loss would decrease only 15% since convection plays a relatively small part at higher environmental conditions. However, at 10°C, a 50% increase in convective loss would eliminate the need for sweating and drop the skin temperature slightly.

An increase in physical effort directly affects heat production, and the partitioning of the energy losses changes correspondingly. An increase in pace to 7 minutes per mile requires an additional 0.6 l/min of oxygen, or a 20% increase in metabolism to 1190 W. The core temperature would rise 0.3°C to about 38.2°C, and the skin temperature would rise slightly by about 0.7°C. The increases in velocity and skin temperature

would increase the convective and radiative losses by only
about 10%. Respiration loss would rise 20% in response to the
increased ventilation. The major effect would be a 210 W increase in evaporative heat transfer required to maintain thermal
equilibrium.

Conclusions

The biophysical relations for energy production in working
muscle have been presented. The various mechanisms by
which energy is transported to the skin are discussed. It is
seen that the major portion of the metabolic energy generated
is thermal energy transported by the blood stream to the skin.
Mechanical work comprises about 20% to this total at most.

The relations governing the transfer of heat from the skin
to the surroundings by convection, radiation, sweat evaporation, and respiration losses are presented. It is seen that the
major modes of heat loss are convection and radiation at low
ambient temperatures, and sweat evaporation at high ambient
temperatures. Changes in environmental conditions alter the
partitioning among these modes, with ambient temperature
having the greatest effect.

References

1. Åstrand, P. O. and K. Rodahl, Testbook of Work Physiol-
    ogy. McGraw Hill, New York, 1970.
2. Bullard, R. W. Physiology of Exercise. In: Physiology,
    E. E. Selkurt, Ed., Little, Brown, and Co., Boston, 1966.
3. Fanger, P. O. Thermal comfort. Danish Technical Press,
    Copenhagen, 1970.
4. McCutchan, F. W., and C. L. Taylor. Respiratory heat
    exchange with varying temperature and humidity of in-
    spired air. J. Appl. Physiol. 31: 121-135, 1951.
5. Mitchell, J. W., E. R. Nadel, and J. A. J. Stolwijk.
    Respiratory weight losses during exercise. J. Appl.Physiol.
    32: 474-476, 1972.
6. Mitchell, J. W., J. A. J. Stolwijk, and E. R. Nadel.
    Model simulation of muscle blood flow and oxygen uptake
    during exercise transients. Biophys. J. 12: 1452-1466,
    1972.

7.   Nishi, Y., and A. P. Gagge. Direct evaluation of convective heat transfer coefficient by napthalene sublimation. J. Appl. Physiol. 29: 830-838, 1970.

8.   "Proposed Standard System of Symbols for Thermal Physiology," J. Appl. Physiol. 27: 439-446, 1969.

9.   Saltin, B., and L. Hermansen. Esophageal, rectal, and muscle temperature during exercise. J. Appl. Physiol. 21: 1757-1762, 1966.

10.   Stolwijk, J. A. J. A mathematical model of physiological temperature regulation in man. NASA Dept. CR-1855, 1971.

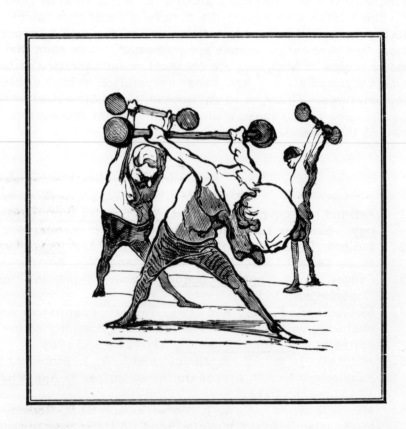

Control of Sweating Rate and
Skin Blood Flow During Exercise

George L. Brengelmann

Introduction: Body Temperature During Exercise

A brief review of the behavior of body temperature during
exercise seems an appropriate introduction to the discussion
of how the effector mechanisms which adjust thermal balance
during exercise are controlled. Internal temperature (non-
specific references to internal temperature will be referred to
as T_c) typically stabilizes at an elevated level during exercise.
This phenomenon is frequently described as temperature regulation about an "elevated set point".

The concept of an elevated set point and controversy about
it date back to the publication of Marius Nielsen's monumen-
tal work (18). Nielsen showed that exercising man exhibits a
stable elevated rectal temperature (T_{re}) throughout long periods
of exercise. The higher the workload, the higher the maintained temperature. Nielsen also showed that this elevated
temperature was rather independent of environmental changes;
over a wide range of conditions, only small deviations of T_{re}
above normal were observed. If just a tenth of a degree or so
change in T_c results from several degrees change in environmental temperature, the hypothesis that a thermostatic mechanism has been reset is tempting. Otherwise, why would not
the temperature regulating system take advantage of conditions promoting heat loss in order to return T_c to normal?

Many investigators have confirmed Nielsen's observations.
Measures of T_c other than T_{re} have been used. Tympanic (T_{ty})
or esophageal (T_{es}) temperatures respond much more rapidly
and exhibit the stable elevated level within about 15 min. A
significant advance contributed by Saltin and Hermansen (21)
was the discovery, confirmed by others (7, 29), that the elevation in T_c maintained during exercise was a function of relative

27

rather than absolute workloads. Different individuals at the
same absolute workload exhibited different maintained levels
of T_{es}, but if these individuals exercised at the same per-
centage of their maximal oxygen consumption (same relative
workload), they exhibited virtually identical patterns of T_{es}.

Arguments against the set point hypothesis have been based
on data such as that shown in Figure 1. The different time

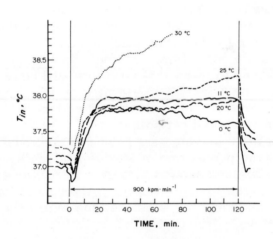

FIG. 1. *Temperature in the lower esophagus dur-*
ing prolonged exercise in various environmental
conditions, with environmental temperatures indi-
cated for each curve. Adapted from Kitzing et al
(12).

courses of T_{re} were obtained in different environmental conditions. Obviously, the temperature maintained during exercise
was influenced by environmental temperature. But, on close
inspection of Nielsen's graphs, which were plotted on a coars-
er scale, one can see that the steady T_{re} levels were also

slightly different with different environmental temperatures.
Wyndham also showed that the maintained T_c varied with environmental temperature (28). Kitzing et al. (12) interpret
this systematic variation with environmental temperature as
evidence that the set point has not been elevated.

The point made by those who argue against a set point
change is that the elevated T_c is merely what is called a load
error. According to this view, body temperature regulation
works as a conventional proportional control system, which
requires an error signal for effector activity. With the onset
of exercise, heat is stored; T_c rises and will continue to do so
until a sufficient signal develops to call for effector activity
adequate to dissipate the large amount of heat produced and
bring about thermal balance -- necessarily at an elevated T_c.
Then, when environmental changes occur, only small changes
in T_c are to be expected since the system presumably has high
gain and will correct for the change with only a small change
in T_c.

A clever approach to this load error question is to vary the
endogenous heat production for the same level of oxygen consumption with "negative" exercise - e.g., walking downhill
or resisting a motor driven bicycle ergometer; situations in
which work done on the subject appears as heat in the exercising muscles. Bodil Nielsen showed that superimposition
of the additional heat produced in negative exercise at a given
oxygen consumption did not elevate T_c above the level associated with positive work at the same oxygen consumption (19).
This would argue against describing the elevated T_c of exercise as a mere load error. However, others who have employed negative work have arrived at conflicting conclusions
(23, 17). Stolwijk and Nadel (23) reported that "neither
exercise per se nor the form of exercise (positive vs. negative
work) presents any exceptions to the regulatory mechanism, as
defined by internal and skin temperature." For a more thorough
treatment of this subject, see the review by Wyndham (27).
Perhaps additional experimental work is needed to resolve this
conflict.

An important fact to bear in mind when studying the litera-
ture on body temperature regulation during exercise is that the
well maintained temperature on which we focus does not pre-
vail in all tissues. An excellent demonstration of this can be
found in the paper of Aikas and co-workers (1). They compared intramuscular temperature with T_{re} and T_{es}. Active

Rs us any

muscle quickly takes on or exceeds the temperature eventually maintained in the esophagus. Inactive muscle, however, exhibited virtually no temperature change during the 15 min bout of exercise except at very high workload. Therefore, when the T_c we measure stabilizes after the first 15 min of exercise, the system is by no means at a steady thermal state. A considerable quantity of tissue is below blood temperature and will gain heat over a long time course. Consider the liver in which blood flow falls during exercise but metabolic rate remains high (20). It is to be expected that temperature in this organ during exercise in the heat could become excessively high with T_{es} or T_{re} still at levels considered tolerable. Two points worth emphasizing, then, are: first, assumptions of thermal steady state during prolonged exercise are likely to be in error—this must be considered in analysis of work which assumes thermal steady state for calculating of tissue conductance during exercise. Second, the temperatures we measure may leave us ignorant of excessively high temperatures in actively metabolizing regions (kidney, liver) with reduced blood flow.

The above brief review of the thermal phenomena which have been observed in exercising man can be summarized as follows: an elevated T_c is maintained within rather narrow limits over a wide range of environmental conditions. This constant temperature does not necessarily represent a steady thermal state because of the relatively slow response of inactive tissues. The phenomenon has been ascribed to a changed set point or to a load error associated with normal temperature regulation, with no clear basis for a choice between the alternatives. Conspicuously lacking are specific definitions of "set point" and "gain".

Modern Approaches to Description of Temperature Regulation During Exercise

A different approach can be seen in recent studies of human temperature regulation in which investigators have attempted to map out the relationship between effector activity and the independent variables which drive the effectors. With this approach, quantitative comparisons of the control of the effectors at rest and during exercise can be made. Questions about "set point" and "gain" can be asked in more specific terms. Ultimately, models of temperature regulation will be developed which incorporate the properties of the effector

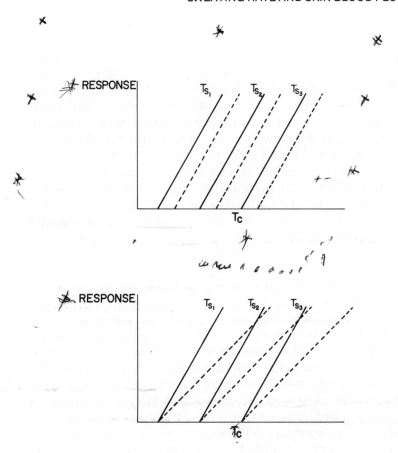

FIG. 2. Results of hypothetical ideal experiments in which response of thermoregulatory
effector (i.e., sweat rate or skin blood flow) is
obtained for wide range of values of skin temperature (T_{s1}, T_{s2}, T_{s3}) and internal temperature,
T_C. Solid lines refer to "data" taken at rest,
dashed lines to "data" taken during a particular
level of exercise. See text for interpretations
of type of results shown in upper panel vs. those
shown in lower panel. Among the requirements for
real experiments to approach this hypothetical
ideal is that the values of the response for a
particular (T_C, T_s) pair are taken at a time when
neither the response, T_C, nor T_s is changing at a
rate such that system sensitivity to rate of change
contributes significantly to the net response.

system and the physical system (see Mitchell et al., [13]). This modern approach can be characterized by the attempt to obtain results whose ideal is shown schematically in Figure 2. T_c and skin temperature (T_s) are regarded as the major independent variables. In the ideal experiment, one would collect values of the effector response over a wide range of values of one of the variables, say T_c, while the other, T_s was held constant. This would be repeated at different values of T_s until completion of a detailed map of the functional relationship. After obtaining such a family of curves in a resting individual, the series of experiments would then be repeated with the individual at each of a range of exercise intensities. The solid lines in the figure represent an hypothetical family of curves found at rest, the dashed lines represent an hypothetical family obtained at some level of exercise. As to interpretation in terms of set point and load error, the upper panel would support a proposal that the elevated T_c maintained during exercise was no more than partly load error, since something which could be described as a set point shift had also occurred. The lower panel would support assertions that not just load error but gain changes were involved. The finding that exactly the same curves were traced in exercise as at rest would unequivocally show that the basic pattern of control is not altered by exercise.

Seasoned investigators will recognize that the above ideal may be rather elusive if not illusive. The practical difficulties of obtaining many lengthy experiments on a single human subject are enormous. A question of reproducibility lurks nearby -- would the subject regenerate the same curve on a subsequent day? How is the acclimatization phenomenon to be dealt with? Can we be sure that a particular value of the effector will be associated with a particular T_c - T_s pair regardless of by what path the values are approached? Nonetheless, various groups have done their best to get as close to the ideal of Figure 2 as possible. First, work on control of sweating (SR) will be discussed, followed by a brief discussion of the relatively small amount of work on the control of skin blood flow (SBF).

Studies of Control of Sweating

A reflection of the ideal of Figure 2 may be seen in Figure 3

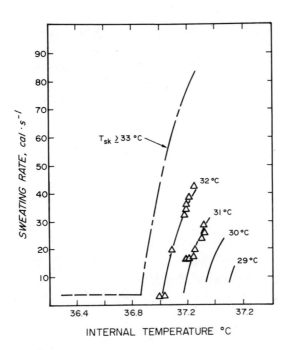

FIG. 3. Rate of sweating vs. tympanic membrane
temperature, from experiments of Benzinger (4).

from Benzinger's work on the control of sweating (4).   To all
appearances, this represents a map of a functional relationship
between SR and T_s and T_{ty}.   According to this description, T_s
has no effect on control of SR if T_s exceeds 33°C.   Below
33°C, T_s systematically suppresses sweating.   Unfortunately,
these data do not establish baseline information about control

of SR during rest to compare with SR responses during exercise. In order to obtain a range of T_s and T_{ty}, Benzinger employed exercise in order to manipulate T_{ty}; for example, to obtain high T_{ty} with a low T_s. Some proportion of these points, then, were obtained during or shortly after exercise. If the low T_s points are the ones obtained with exercise, then perhaps the displacement of the curve is due to exercise, not T_s. Even if the actual data were taken after cessation of exercise, the possibility remains that effects of exercise persisted such that pure "resting" data were not obtained. Also, relying on data taken during transient periods entails dangers of ascribing to T_s and T_c influences which actually are associated with their rates of change or lags in the system response.

Thus, serious questions arise on study of the data in Figure 3. But, all the workers who have sought to provide descriptions of an effector variable in terms of T_s and T_c have had to contend with similar problems simply because the variables cannot be manipulated independently.

Recently, the major work on control of SR patterned after the hypothetical ideal of Figure 2 has been carried out by the investigators associated with the Pierce Foundation Laboratory. They have described control of SR in terms of T_s and T_c (usually measured as T_{es}) and have gone on to study the influence of local T_s and skin wettedness (9, 14, 15, 16, 22). In Chapter 5, Dr. Stolwijk describes the changes brought about in long term processes - repeated heat exposure and exercise. Just how quantitative their efforts have been can be seen from the following equation (Eq. 1) which summarizes their results.

$$E = (197(T_c - 36.7) + 23(\bar{T}_s - 34.0))e^{(\Sigma \bar{T}_{sl} - 34)/10}$$

$$\text{in } W/m^2 \quad (Eq\ 1)$$

where E = evaporative heat loss

$\bar{T}_{sl}$ = mean weighted local skin temperatures

Figure 4 shows some of their experimental data with lines calculated from their model.

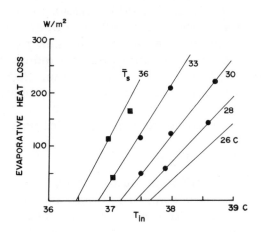

FIG. 4.   *Rate of evaporation of sweat vs. internal temperature (measured in the esophagus or at the tympanum), from Nadel et al (14), with permission of the American Physiological Society.   Solid lines calculated from Eq. 1.   Filled squares are data points taken at rest, filled circles are data points taken during exercise.   The authors emphasized that these are steady state points.*

The authors state that this relationship has been tested and has fit widely varying conditions with and without exercise. Exercise was used to bring about increases in T_C but, according to these authors, no effect is seen of exercise <u>per se.</u> Presumably, they arrive at particular pairs of T_C and T_S by different routes so that they could conclude that the response associated with a particular pair was independent of the path by which it was approached.

Data obtained in our laboratory, limited to the control of SR
in resting man, basically confirms the above results except
that we have found relatively greater influence of T_c and less
of T_s (30). We also found non-linear characteristics at high
T_s (31).

At present, then, one must conclude from the best available
evidence that control of SR during exercise is the same as at
rest. However, Dr. Nadel would be among the first to point
out that it is not yet time to discard our sweat capsules or to
rely on the above equation as a complete description of how
sweating is regulated. Additional work is required, particularly in the area of transients. For example, Nadel et al. as
well as others (14, 26) have pointed out that negative rate of
change of T_s can act as a powerful inhibitor of SR, but this
variable is not yet incorporated in the model of Eq. 1.

Control of Skin Blood Flow

Relatively little work in pursuit of the goals of Figure 2 has
been published on the control of skin blood flow (SBF). Most
of the efforts at quantitative resolution of control in terms of
T_c and T_s have been carried out in our laboratory (10, 11, 30,
31) and by a group of investigators at the Pierce Foundation
(24, 25).

Before work in this area could proceed, an adequate method
for SBF measurement in supine or upright man at rest and at
work had to be found. Some investigators in the field of temperature regulation with similar goals used whole body conductance -- heat loss divided by the difference between T_c and T_s
-- as the measure of SBF (3). Interpretations based on whole
body conductance are necessarily severely limited because (i)
at best this is an operational definition of that blood flow necessary to supply the observed heat loss if blood arrived at the
skin at T_c and left at T_s, and (ii) it is inappropriate for use
with T_s defined as the area-weighted average of temperatures
from multiple sites (6). Also, as pointed out above, steady
states in which heat production equals heat loss do not occur
until long after the establishment of apparently stable T_c
measured as T_{es}, T_{ty}, etc., so that computations of conductance based on heat production are likely to be greatly in
error.

Cardiovascular physiologists who have studied the

cutaneous circulation in man have typically used venous
occlusion plethysmography for measurements of forearm blood
flow (FBF). Changes in SBF can be inferred from changes in
FBF provided that flow to underlying muscle (MBF) remains
constant. A long series of investigations have established
that MBF is not increased by either direct or indirect heating
under a variety of conditions (see summary in 8, 11). A decrease in MBF is sometimes found, but is small compared to
total change in SBF. It is generally assumed that forearm skin
is representative of skin over the major proportion of the body
surface excluding acral regions in which active vasodilation
is not found.

Adaptation of venous occlusion plethysmography to use in
exercising man proved a difficult problem since movement of
the arm produces large artifacts. Our laboratory and Wenger
et al. independently achieved means of stabilizing the forearm
during exercise. Up to moderate levels of exercise, virtually
artifact-free records can be obtained (10, 11).

Another basic problem encountered in studies of the relative
roles of T_c and T_s in control of SBF is what to do about local
temperature. If T_s is to be driven to 38°C or above, a local
effect is to be expected. If the forearm alone is heated to 38°C
or above, FBF increases progressively with time, reaching a
peak in 40 min or more (2). The effect increases with local T_s
and is quite variable among individuals both in time course and
degree of elevation of FBF. Thus, if FBF is recorded from a
portion of the forearm which is held at the same temperature as
T_s, i.e., the temperature of the remainder of the body skin,
then the flow measured must be thought of as under the influence of local temperature as well as T_s and T_c. The local
effect can be expected to increase generally with time. We
have compared FBF measured in one arm kept at neutral temperatures, e.g., 32°C, with FBF in the other arm held at a temperature high enough to produce a local effect. In general, the
difference can be described as indicating a superimposition of
the local effect upon a pure "reflex" response, i.e., that observed in the neutral arm, but clearly not a simple additive
combination of the two influences. We and others (24) have
assumed that studies of reflex control should begin with temperature of the forearm held low enough to avoid an appreciable
local effect. Unless otherwise indicated, the studies mentioned henceforth were done with local forearm temperature at
36°C or less.

Studies of SBF Control at Rest

In two studies of control of SBF in supine resting men, Wyss et al. reported findings which have important bearing on the subject of control during exercise beyond their value as baseline data on control at rest (30, 31). Wyss et al. controlled T_s with water-perfused suits. They drove T_s in different temporal patterns to aid in separation of T_c and T_s contributions to the SBF responses. Two different measures of T_c were used, T_{es} and right atrial temperature (T_{ra}). The latter responds more rapidly to changes in thermal balance. Results were described in terms of a linear combination of T_s and T_c. The regression analysis yielded coefficients for T_c and T_s with a ratio of roughly 10:1 when T_{es} was used as the measure of T_c. But, with T_{ra} used for T_c, this ratio was 20:1 or more. These results emphasize the problem of interpreting data taken during transient periods. If responses to an increase in T_c brought about by T_s elevation are analyzed, the longer the time lag in the particular measure of T_c chosen, the greater the apparent influence of T_s. If T_{re} were used as the measure of T_c in certain protocols, all the response would have to be ascribed to T_s since little or no change in T_{re} may develop during a 10 or 15 minute period of increasing FBF following increase in T_s.

Wyss et al. also pointed out pitfalls of the regression technique and emphasized that the contribution of T_s at high T_s appears to be quite non-linear. Linear regression analysis assumes the variables interact linearly and will produce misleading parameters to the extent that the variables actually interact non-linearly.

Studies of SBF Control During Exercise

In the past, FBF has been recorded in supine men during brief periods of mild exercise (5). These were studies oriented toward cardiovascular control rather than thermoregulation. Vasoconstriction of both skin and muscle in the forearm occurred with the onset of exercise followed thereafter by increase in SBF along with T_c with MBF remaining low and constant. Johnson and Rowell (11) verified this pattern in upright men exercising at moderate levels.

The background of knowledge in cardiovascular physiology offers the clear implication that control of SBF should in fact be modified during exercise. The skin is not the sole property of thermoregulation; as demands for flow elsewhere increase, SBF may well be reduced in compensation. Furthermore, the adjustment to the volume redistributions associated with changes in posture can be expected to alter SBF (see Chapter 4). Therefore, pursuit of the ideal of Figure 2 requires that we also systematically vary the variables of exercise and posture, greatly complicating an already complex experimental undertaking.

First steps have been taken by Wenger et al. and Johnson et al. with different experimental designs. The approach of Wenger et al. was to obtain the SBF-T_{es} relationship at three different relative workloads for two levels of body T_s obtained by varying environmental conditions (24). They reported that FBF increased linearly with T_{es} for a given T_s and that this relationship was shifted to the right with decreasing T_s, i.e., reduced T_s had the effect of inhibiting flow for a given T_{es}. They found that workload did not alter the relationships. The ratio of change in FBF to change in T_{es} was roughly 6-7 flow units per °C.

Johnson et al. used a different experimental strategy. They compared responses at rest and during work at both the upright and supine posture (10) but did not vary workload. They used the same level of T_s in all experiments to avoid the complication of dealing with still another variable. The level of T_s chosen was 38°C. This elevated level was necessary in order to obtain sufficient increases in T_{es}. Figure 5 shows their results. We believe that these results show clearly that control of FBF is radically altered during exercise, at least at this T_s and the moderate levels of exercise of short duration employed. For the same T_{es} and with T_s at 38°C, much lower flow is supplied to skin in an exercising man than in a man at supine rest. The ratio of change in FBF to change in T_{es} found in upright exercise was roughly the same as that found by Wenger et al.

The results of Johnson et al. may appear to conflict with those of Wenger et al. if the implication is drawn from the latter work that the independence of workload between 30 and 70 per cent can be extrapolated to suggest that the independence extends to zero workload, i.e., rest. Another extrapolation which produces a conflict would be to draw from the findings of Wenger et al. the inference that the results of Johnson et al. can be extrapolated to lower levels of T_s in the physiological range of exercise with only a displacement of the

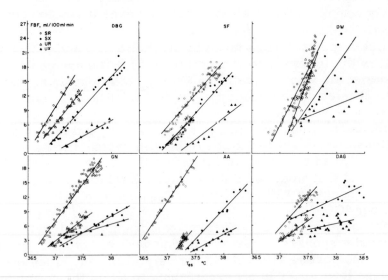

FIG. 5. *Forearm blood flow vs. T_{es} in six subjects studied under four conditions: supine rest (open circles), supine exercise (filled circles), upright rest (open triangles), and upright exercise (filled triangles). All these data were obtained with T_s at 38°C. In protocols which included exercise, T_s was stabilized at 38°C before exercise began. The solid lines are least-squares best fits. From Johnson et al (10), with permission of the American Physiological Society.*

FBF-T_{es} curve along the T_{es} axis, preserving the marked difference between patterns of response at supine rest, upright exercise, etc. This extrapolation would produce a conflict with the findings of Wyss et al. on the relative ratios of sensitivity to T_s and T_c at rest. Clearly, further experimental verification and extension of both sets of experiments is needed. We feel it is particularly important to work out how independence of workload is compatible with the indications that sympathetic vasoconstrictor activity increases in proportion to exercise activity (see following chapter).

We have attempted two approaches to the problem of studying the FBF-T_{es} relationship during exercise in a different range of T_s. In the first, FBF was simply monitored during prolonged upright exercise with the lightly clad subject exposed in a neutral environment. T_s remained within approximately 30 to 32°C. Flow increased very little until the stable level of T_{es} was reached; thereafter, FBF increased at virtually constant T_{es}. Figure 6 shows the typical FBF-T_{es} pattern

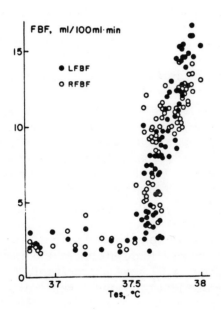

Fig. 6. Forearm blood flow measured in the left arm (filled circles) and right arm (open circles) vs. T_{es} during prolonged exercise (60 min). The subject wore only shorts. The air-conditioned room was at 21°C. From Johnson et al (11), with permission of the American Physiological Society.

observed. The lowest slope observed was 25 flow units per °C, higher than coefficients reported by Wenger et al. and actually higher than values reported by Wyss et al. for resting man. However, final levels of FBF observed were less than levels previously observed for the same T_C at rest, a finding interpreted to support the earlier conclusion that FBF at a given T_{es} is attenuated by exercise. Johnson et al. questioned whether the presentation of data as in Figure 6 was misleading in its implication that T_{es} was the drive for the FBF response, and suggested that lagging temperatures from other thermosensitive sites may have been important in driving the response.

The second approach was to begin exercise with a controlled low T_S and, after establishment of stable T_{es}, drive T_S rapidly to 38°C, the level at which the data of Figure 5 were obtained. Figure 7 shows typical results. The stepwise elevation in T_S was typically accompanied by a transient fall in T_{es} during which FBF rose. Thereafter, T_{es} rose but with little further increase in FBF. These findings contrast markedly with those described in the previous paragraph. On comparison of Figures 6 and 7, the inference can be drawn that the higher level of T_S actually has the effect of inhibiting flow increase.

Finally, we have extended our observations of the FBF-T_{es} relationship with T_S held at 38°C to observe the time course of FBF with longer periods of exercise than used in the experiments of Figure 5. The typical response pattern is shown in Figure 8. Most subjects exhibited a saturation in response, i.e., with exercise in the heat prolonged, T_{es} continued to increase, but FBF reached a plateau just beyond the degree of elevation shown in Figure 5.

We cannot conclude at this point whether the pattern of Figure 6 or that of Figure 8 accurately represents the pattern of control in the range of T_S over which stable T_{es} will be maintained during moderate levels of exercise. Either represents a departure from the pattern of control at rest, but the pattern of Figure 8 would be described as a much attenuated sensitivity to change in T_c, and that of Figure 6 actually as a heightened sensitivity attained only after an elevated T_C threshold is reached. The former pattern would be associated with relatively poor regulation of T_C during exercise about an elevated level largely the result of load error. The latter would be associated with regulation superior to that at rest, i.e., greater FBF response to a given perturbation in T_c, with a large proportion of the elevation in T_{es} due to the increase in

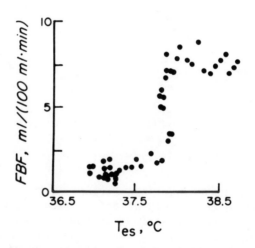

FIG. 7. *Forearm blood flow vs. T_{es} in an exercising subject with T_s driven from 32°C to 38°C after T_{es} stabilized. The initial horizontal portion of the relationship and a slight initial upturn was traced as the subject exercised with a cool skin and T_{es} rose. The nearly vertical portion of the curve followed when T_s was then driven rapidly to 38°C, i.e., FBF rose rapidly with T_s at nearly constant T_{es}. Thereafter, T_{es} increased with little further FBF increase as exercise continued with T_s at 38°C.*

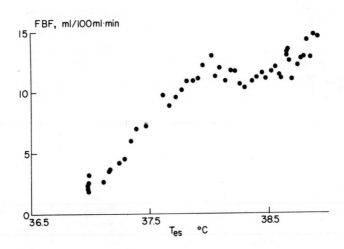

FIG. 8. Forearm blood flow vs. T_{es} during exercise with T_s held at 38°C. Protocol was identical to that described as "upright exercise" in
Figure 5, i.e., T_s was driven to 38°C before
exercise commerced, but the period of exercise
at T_s 38°C was extended to investigate whether
FBF would continue to increase in proportion
to T_{es} at higher levels of T_{es}. Note the
plateau in the response.

the threshold T_C level below which no FBF elevation is seen.

Future attempts to clarify quantitative understanding of SBF control will require overcoming difficulties which should be mentioned before concluding this discussion. They fall into two categories.

First, we have the problems associated with obtaining steady-state data. A man exercising in a neutral or cool environment, for example, will not exhibit a full range of T_c change at constant T_s; he approaches a stable T_c quickly in a transient period in which both T_s and T_c are changing. Thus, we do not obtain steady-state points for a range of (T_s, T_c) pairs. Given the presence of sensitivity to rate of change of the controlling variables in other effector systems of thermoregulation, we should be alert to the possibility that lead and lag terms are required for description of dynamic characteristics of SBF responses.

The second category is the large area of problems with reproducibility. We have treated problems in this category as due to a variable or variables we do not understand; possibly hormonal, possibly related to heat storage in regions in which temperature lags behind T_{es}. As an example, we have on several occasions attempted to proceed with a second protocol after a subject has completed a period of exercise or heating followed by an intervening rest period long enough for T_{es} to return to control. These subjects exhibited much higher flows for the same T_c and T_s in a subsequent period of warming and/ or exercise (10). Another problem in this category is effects of the acclimatization process. We have attempted to minimize the effects of previous exposure by separating experimental sessions by at least one week. Yet we have seen differences of more than $0.5°C$ in threshold T_{es} in identical protocols performed more than one week apart. Others have evidently not experienced similar difficulties. Although Wenger et al. mentioned that they performed more than one run on the same day, they have not mentioned problems in reproducing the same FBF-T_{es} relationship.

Thus, we see FBF as a function also of recent history and possible other variables not reflected in what we interpret as our independent variables; T_c, T_{es}, posture and level of exercise. These problems can be expected to yield a large ratio of biological noise to biological signal. We expect they will continue to plague us and that our picture of the control of SBF will be clouded by noise and by the particular pathways of travel on the T_c - T_s plane to which we are limited. A clear need is for experiments directed simply at obtaining a measure of the reproducibility which can be obtained in a carefully repeated set of experiments with identical protocol. We do not understand why studies on control of sweating have not been troubled by similar problems if that is, in fact, the correct inference to be drawn from the mathematical descriptions which have been published. We feel that experimental verification of the variability to be expected in this control mechanism is also required.

References

1. Aikas, E., M.J. Karvonen, P. Piironen, and R. Ruosteenoja. Intramuscular, rectal and oesophageal temperature during exercise. Acta Physiol. Scand. 54:366-370, 1962.
2. Barcroft, H., and O. G. Edholm. The effect of temperature on blood flow and deep temperature in the human forearm. J. Physiol., London 102: 5-20, 1943.
3. Benzinger, T. H. Heat regulation: homeostasis of central temperature in man. Physiol. Rev. 49: 672-759, 1969.
4. Benzinger, T. H. The diminution of thermoregulatory sweating during cold-reception at the skin. Proc. Natl. Acad. Sci. 47: 1683-1688, 1961.
5. Bevegård, B. S., and J. T. Shepherd. Regulation of the circulation during exercise in man. Physiol. Rev. 47: 178-213, 1967.
6. Brown, A. C., and G. L. Brengelmann. The interaction of peripheral and central inputs in the temperature regulation system. In: Physiological and Behavioral Temperature Regulation, edited by J. D. Hardy, A. P. Gagge, and J. A. J. Stolwijk. Springfield, Ill., Charles C. Thomas, 1970.
7. Davies, C. T. M., C. Barnes, and A. J. Sargeant. Body temperature in exercise: effects of acclimatization to heat and habituation to work. Intern. Z. Angew. Physiol. 30: 10-19, 1971.
8. Detry, J.-M.R., G. L. Brengelmann, L. B. Rowell, and C. Wyss. Skin and muscle components of forearm blood flow in directly heated resting man. J. Appl. Physiol. 32: 506-511, 1972.
9. Hardy, J. D., and J. A. J. Stolwijk. Partitional calorimetric studies of man during exposures to thermal transients. J. Appl. Physiol. 21: 1799-1806, 1966.
10. Johnson, J. M., L. B. Rowell, and G. L. Brengelmann. Modification of the skin blood flow-body temperature relationship by upright exercise. J. Appl. Physiol. 37: 880-886, 1974.

11. Johnson, J. M., and L. B. Rowell. Forearm skin and muscle vascular responses to prolonged leg exercise in man. J. Appl. Physiol. 39: 920-924, 1975.
12. Kitzing, J., D. Kutta, and A. Bleichert. Temperaturregulation bei langdauernder schwerer körperlicher Arbeit. Pflugers Arch. 301: 241-253, 1968.
13. Mitchell, D., A. R. Atkins, and C. H. Wyndham. Mathematical and physical models of thermoregulation. In: Essays on Temperature Regulation, edited by J. Bligh and R. Moore. North-Holland Publishing Company, Amsterdam, London, 1972, p. 37-54.
14. Nadel, E. R., R. W. Bullard, and J. A. J. Stolwijk. Importance of skin temperature in the regulation of sweating. J. Appl. Physiol. 31: 80-87, 1971.
15. Nadel, E. R., J. W. Mitchell, B. Saltin, and J. A. J. Stolwijk. Peripheral modifications to the central drive for sweating. J. Appl. Physiol. 31: 828-833, 1971.
16. Nadel, E. R., and J. A. J. Stolwijk. Effect of skin wettedness on sweat gland function. Biometerology 5: 87-88, 1972.
17. Nadel, E. R., U. Bergh, and B. Saltin. Body temperatures during negative work exercise. J. Appl. Physiol. 33: 553-558, 1972.
18. Nielsen, M. Die Regulation der Korpertemperatur bei Muskelarbeit. Skand. Arch. Physiol. 79: 193-230, 1938.
19. Nielsen, B. Regulation of body temperature and heat dissipation at different levels of energy- and heat production in man. Acta Physiol. Scand. 68: 215-227, 1966.
20. Rowell, L. B., G. L. Brengelmann, J. R. Blackmon, R. D. Twiss, and F. Kusumi. Splanchnic blood flow and metabolism in heat-stressed man. J. Appl. Physiol. 4: 475-484, 1968.
21. Saltin, B., and L. Hermansen. Esophageal, rectal, and muscle temperature during exercise. J. Appl. Physiol. 21: 1757-1762, 1966.
22. Stolwijk, J. A. J., and J. D. Hardy. Partial calorimetric studies of the thermoregulatory responses of man to thermal transients. J. Appl. Physiol. 21: 966-977, 1966.
23. Stolwijk, J. A. J., and E. R. Nadel. Thermoregulation during positive and negative work exercise. Fed. Proc. 32: 1607-1613, 1973.

24. Wenger, C. B., M. F. Roberts, J. A. J. Stolwijk, and E. R. Nadel. Forearm blood flow during body temperature transients produced by leg exercise. J. Appl. Physiol. 38: 58-63, 1975.
25. Wenger, C. B., M. F. Roberts, E. R. Nadel, and J. A. J. Stolwijk. Thermoregulatory control of finger blood flow. J. Appl. Physiol. 38: 1078-1082, 1975.
26. Wurster, R. D., and R. D. McCook. Influence of rate of change in skin temperature on sweating. J. Appl. Physiol. 27: 237-240, 1969.
27. Wyndham, C. H. The physiology of exercise under heat stress. Ann. Rev. Physiol. 35: 193-220, 1973.
28. Wyndham, C. H., N. B. Strydom, J. F. Morrison, F. D. du Tout, and J. G. Kraan. Responses of unacclimatized men under stress of heat and work. J. Appl. Physiol. 6: 681-686, 1954.
29. Wyndham, C. H., N. B. Strydom, A. J. Van Resnburg, and G. G. Rogers. Effects on maximal oxygen intake of acute changes in altitude in a deep mine. J. Appl. Physiol. 29: 552-555, 1970.
30. Wyss, C. R., G. L. Brengelmann, J. M. Johnson, L. B. Rowell, and M. Niederberger. Control of skin blood flow, sweating and heart rate: role of skin vs. core temperature. J. Appl. Physiol. 36: 726-733, 1974.
31. Wyss, C. R., G. L. Brengelmann, J. M. Johnson, L. B. Rowell, and D. Silverstein. Altered control of skin blood flow at high skin and core temperatures. J. Appl. Physiol. 38: 839-845, 1975.

Competition Between Skin and Muscle
for Blood Flow During Exercise

Loring B. Rowell

The title of this chapter implies that a competition exists between skin and muscle for the available blood supply during exercise. The central question dealt with in this chapter is why such a competition exists even when the exercise imposes well below maximal demands for both oxygen transport and cardiac output. Why is the demand for increased skin blood flow not met simply by a rise in cardiac output until either an adequate skin blood flow is achieved or a maximal cardiac output is reached? Such a scheme, illustrated in Fig. 1, was once proposed by Brouha (5) but is now known not

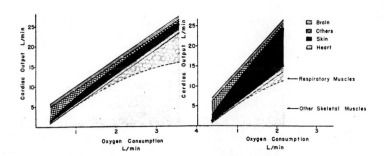

FIG. 1. *Hypothetical scheme for distribution of blood flow during exercise in cool (left panel) and hot environments (right panel). The skin blood flow (shown as the darkened region) could be increased to meet thermoregulatory demands by marked elevations in cardiac output at a given $\dot{V}_{O_2}$ during exercise. Elevations in skin blood flow were expected to drive cardiac output to its maximal value at submaximal $\dot{V}_{O_2}$. (Modified from Brouha [5].)*

to happen. As we shall see, skin and muscle indeed do compete for blood flow during exercise. Why?

The answer appears to lie in upright man's difficulty in
dealing with shifts in blood volume. Normally, blood pressure can be well maintained or increased during exercise
despite massive vasodilation in skeletal muscle. Normal
man has little difficulty in correcting for vasodilation in skeletal muscle, for example, by a combination of increased
cardiac output and regional vasoconstriction. One should
note, however, that despite the very high blood flow in vasodilated skeletal muscle, there is little increase in muscle
blood volume (2). In contrast, man does have great difficulty
in counteracting the shifts in blood volume that attend vasodilation in highly compliant and capacious regions such as the
skin. Thus, a rise in skin blood flow appears to be associated with a marked increase in cutaneous venous volume (27,
28, 38, 42).

In this chapter, we will examine step by step the hemody-
namic consequences of cutaneous vasodilation and the overall
cardiovascular adjustments that are elicited. As a starting
point, it is instructive to examine the range of skin blood
flow of man in <u>supine</u> posture, a position in which hydrostatic forces on distribution of blood volume are minimal.

Fig. 2 illustrates the results from 12 men whose entire
bodies were subjected to direct heating until they reached
their subjective limits of thermal tolerance, without thermal
pain (27). Body skin temperature (T_s) was held at approximately 40°C until right atrial blood temperature (T_{ra}) reached
from 39 to 39.5°C. The rationale of this approach was to
determine the "maximal" response of skin blood flow to combined reflex and local effects of heat. Cardiac output rose
6.6 L/min, and forearm blood flow (FBF) increased six-fold.
The six-fold increase in FBF represents an 11-fold increase
in forearm skin blood flow (from 2 to 22 ml/min per 100 ml of
forearm). Forearm muscle blood flow, which is about one
half of the total FBF, or 2 ml/min per 100 ml of forearm,
remains constant during heat stress (3, 8, 10, 25). Since
blood flow to other major vascular beds, such as renal and
splanchnic, falls, the increase in cardiac output must go to
the skin. If we add what is redistributed from other regions,
then skin blood flow can reach 7 to 8 L/min during or near
maximal vasodilation. As we shall see, such increases in

cardiac output and FBF far exceed those seen at similar or higher body core temperatures (T_c) during upright exercise.

Let us turn now to a far more complex problem: how does the cardiovascular system adjust to increases in skin blood flow and skin blood volume when man is upright? As Amberson said (1), "when man's subhuman ancestors dared to rise and

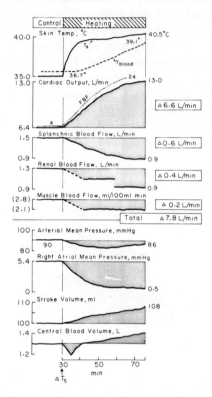

FIG. 2. *Average circulatory changes in subjects directly heated by maintenance of body T_S at 40 to 41°C. Initial and final values and time course are shown for T_S, right atrial blood temperature, and each cardiovascular variable. Contributions of increased cardiac output and reduced regional blood flows to total skin blood flow (7.8 L/min) are shown in the boxes on the right. All data except splanchnic blood flow (7 men) and renal blood flow (1 man plus data of Radigan and Robinson [24]) and atrial pressure (4 men) are averaged from 12 to 17 men. (From Rowell [27], by permission of the American Physiological Society.)*

walk upon their hind legs, they essayed a physiological experiment of no mean difficulty". Seventy percent of the total
blood volume is below the heart in upright man, and 80 percent of this volume is in distensible veins. Dependent veins
are subjected to the fully hydrostatic effect of the continuous
column of blood between them and the heart once they have
filled and their valves are open. The amount of blood that
they hold depends upon the hydrostatic pressure (i.e., their
distance below the heart) and their compliance ($\Delta v/\Delta p$).
Matters are made even worse for the heated man by an increase in skin venous compliance with heating. As the data
in Fig. 3 show, the volume of blood held in the legs at a
given pressure increases with increasing leg T_s (increased
skin venous compliance). If we take 50 mm Hg as an average

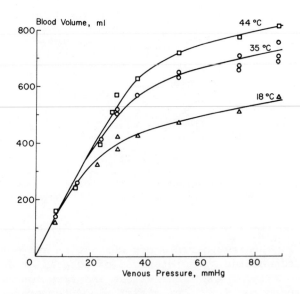

FIG. 3. *Relationship between venous pressure in
leg veins and the volume of blood contained at
three different bath temperatures. Increased
temperature increases the volume of blood contained in veins at a given distending pressure
(increased venous compliance $\Delta v/\Delta p$). Redrawn
from Gauer and Thorn [3].*

venous distending pressure between the heart and feet in upright posture (it would be 90 to 100 mm Hg at the feet), then
leg volume would increase 200 to 250 ml with increased leg
T_s. It is common knowledge that humans heated to the degree illustrated in Fig. 2 cannot stand without fainting
rapidly (21).

The large shift of volume into the skin has profound effects
on the central circulation. These effects are schematically
illustrated in Fig. 4. While cutaneous venous volume increases, return of blood to the heart decreases proportionally.

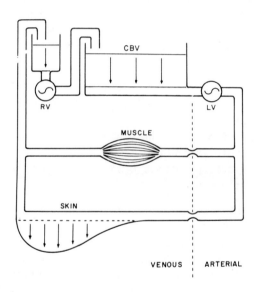

FIG. 4. *Schematic illustration of effects of skin
vasodilation upon central vascular volume. As
skin veins fill, the venous return is temporarily
reduced so that preventricular volume sumps are
depleted (see text).*

Unless volume is displaced centrally from dependent veins by movement of the legs or by venoconstriction, the right and left ventricular outputs could only be transiently maintained at a given level by depletion of their preventricular sumps or "reservoirs". The pulmonary region (labelled CBV in Fig. 4) is the sump for the left ventricle (LV), and the thoracic veins and probably splanchnic veins are volume sumps for the right ventricle (RV). The fall in central venous pressure and splanchnic vasoconstriction both act to displace passively the blood volume from the splanchnic region by reducing splanchnic venous distension. Thus, when the skin vasodilates and its veins fill, the right ventricle rapidly depletes its volume sumps, and central venous pressure and right ventricular filling pressure fall. The left ventricle withdraws blood volume from the pulmonary vessels (shown as decreased central blood volume [CBV] in Fig. 4) that cannot be refilled by the volume-depleted right ventricle. Thus, we see the following responses to vasodilation of the skin in upright man:

i) decreased thoracic blood volume,
ii) decreased central venous pressure and ventricular filling pressure,
iii) decreased stroke volume and decreased cardiac output despite increased heart rate, and
iv) decreased arterial blood pressure despite visceral vasoconstriction.

Under conditions of maximal skin vasodilation, shown in Fig. 2, if man stood up, stroke volume and cardiac output would fall so drastically that blood pressure would drop precipitously and syncope would ensue. We all know that man can tolerate some heat stress in upright posture; however, the time to syncope is less than what it would be, for example, during a head-up tilt in cool conditions. The question is how the circulation adjusts in man so that he can stand up and exercise under varying degrees of hyperthermia. The simplest solution would be to constrict the dilated cutaneous veins when blood pressure and central venous pressure fall. The venoconstriction would rapidly return blood volume to the thorax and restore central venous pressure, stroke volume, cardiac output, and blood pressure. In upright resting man, this adjustment does not occur; veins of skin and skeletal muscle are not targets of baroreceptor mediated reflexes (28, 39).

Man's key line of defense against heat syncope is vasocon-

striction, not venoconstriction, of the skin. This point is of
central importance in understanding how upright man adjusts to
heat stress and exercise. By vasoconstricting the skin, man
reduces the rate at which dependent cutaneous veins fill (16).
Of course, these veins will eventually fill up; the final volume
will depend upon their distance below the heart (hydrostatic
component) and their compliance (increased somewhat by heating). Fainting will then ensue, unless there is movement of
the legs. The importance of movement is described below.
The magnitude and significance of skin vasoconstriction are
illustrated in Fig. 5. In this example, the investigators

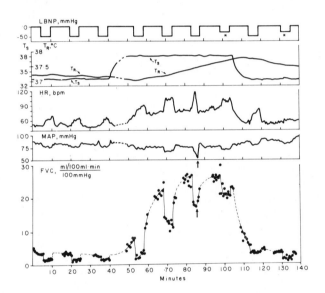

FIG. 5. Skin vasoconstriction in response to lower
body negative pressure (LBNP) in heat-stressed
man. The top panel shows when 5-min periods of
LBNP were applied before and after whole body T_s
(second panel) was raised so as to increase body
temperature (T_r, second panel) and increase forearm skin vascular conductance (FVC, bottom panel).
Note the arrow at 85 min and the marked fall in
mean arterial pressure (MAP, fourth panel).
This subject could no longer elicit sufficient
skin vasoconstriction to overcome syncope.
(From Johnson et al. [16], by permission of the
American Physiological Society.)

directly heated the subjects by raising body T_s to 38°C for 65 min while applying lower body negative pressure (LBNP) at -50 mm Hg below the iliac crest for 5 of each 15 min (16). This stress is roughly equivalent to a 90° head-up tilt. With each application of LBNP, the skin vasoconstricted markedly, but skin blood flow was still well above control levels. Ultimately, a point was reached where vasoconstriction was not sufficient to prevent a major decrease in blood pressure (note the arrow in Fig. 5). Fainting was averted by a release of the suction on the legs. If all of the values for forearm skin vascular conductance (i.e., skin blood flow normalized for blood pressure changes) are plotted, we see in Fig. 6 that skin blood flow is

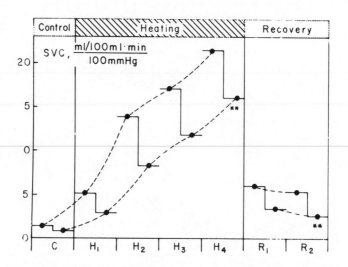

FIG. 6. *Skin vascular conductance (SVC) during control period with body T_s normal and during whole body heating (T_s, 38°C) (H_1-H_4) and recovery. The top dashed line indicates average SVC from 3 men before LBNP was applied (a constant forearm muscle vascular conductance was subtracted). The lower dashed line shows average SVC for these 3 subjects when LBNP was applied. One would expect similar curves were SVC compared in men heated at supine vs. upright rest (see reference 18). (From Johnson et al. [16], by permission of the American Physiological Society.)*

much lower at a given skin and core temperature when man is stressed by gravity (or LBNP) than when he is not. Others have made similar or related observations using different experimental approaches (7, 21, 22, 23).

When upright man begins to exercise, the situation changes. First, exercise appears to be an added stimulus to cutaneous vasoconstriction. This point is discussed by Brengelmann (6) in Chapter 3 (see Fig. 5) of this book and is based upon evidence from Johnson et al. (18). Cutaneous venous filling rates will be even lower at a given T_C during upright exercise than during upright rest. Also, muscle contraction helps to empty cutaneous veins so that the _average_ venous volume decreases.

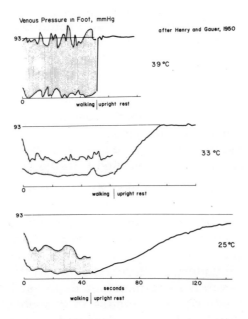

FIG. 7. *Changes in pressure in veins of the foot during walking at three ambient temperatures. Exercise always caused rapid venous emptying, but as venous filling rate increased with rising temperature owing to dilation of skin arterioles, average venous pressure, and thus venous volume, rose. Note the effects of temperature on the venous filling rate when exercise stopped. Redrawn from Henry and Gauer [15].*

Henry and Gauer's (15) work (Fig. 7) illustrates the emptying
and filling of veins in the foot with each step during exercise.
In cool environments (25°C) the veins fill so slowly that the
average venous pressure remains well below the full hydrostatic pressure. Note how slowly the veins fill when exercise stops. In warmer conditions (33°C, Fig. 7), the veins
fill faster so that average venous pressure, and thus average
venous volume, is higher. Note how much more rapidly the
veins fill when exercise ceases. In hot environments (39°C),
average venous pressure is most markedly increased during
exercise and veins fill most rapidly when exercise stops.
These experiments indicate that even during exercise average
venous pressure and volume will be greater when the skin is
vasodilated than when it is not.

It follows from the foregoing comments that a rise in skin
blood flow during prolonged exercise should be accompanied
by some of the changes schematically outlined in Fig. 4.
In fact, Ekelund (11) found the following changes attending
prolonged exercise in cool (20 to 24°C) environments (Fig. 8):

   i) a progressive fall in stroke volume,
  ii) a progressive fall in central venous pressure
       and pulmonary arterial pressure,
 iii) a progressive fall in arterial blood pressure, and
  iv) a constant cardiac output and a rising heart rate.

These data suggest that a progressive rise in skin blood
flow and skin blood volume occurs throughout exercise. This
notion was tested under similar conditions by Johnson and
Rowell (17) and forearm skin blood flow did rise progressively
through prolonged, moderately heavy exercise (Fig. 9). The
blood flow to the underlying forearm skeletal muscle decreased
at the onset of exercise and remained depressed thereafter;
thus, the exercise-induced increase in vasoconstrictor outflow
to inactive skeletal muscle is maintained or increased throughout exercise just as it is to splanchnic and renal vascular
beds (27).

By suddenly changing T_s and then clamping it at high or low
levels, investigators (34) were able to exaggerate or prevent
the "cardiovascular drift" described by Ekelund. Through the
use of water-perfused suits, T_s was held near 32°C for 30 min
(control period) and then raised to 38°C during the next 30 min
as illustrated in Fig. 10 (34). As we can see, "cardiovascular
drift" occurred during the first 30 min of exercise while body

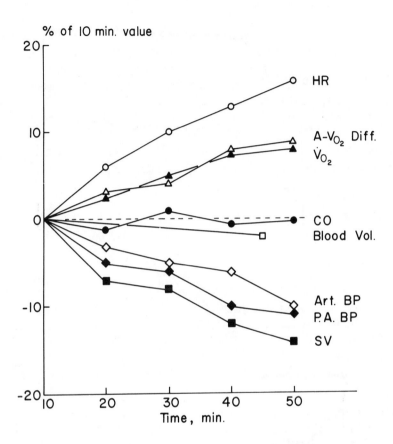

FIG. 8. Circulatory responses to prolonged exercise in a neutral (20°C) environment. Gradual vasodilation of skin (see Fig. 9) causes a progressive downward "drift" in arterial blood pressure (Art. BP) and pulmonary arterial pressure (P.A.BP), with decreased stroke volume (SV), compensated for by rising heart rate (HR) while cardiac output (CO) stays constant. The decline of pressures was not caused by reduced blood volume. (Redrawn from Ekelund [11].)

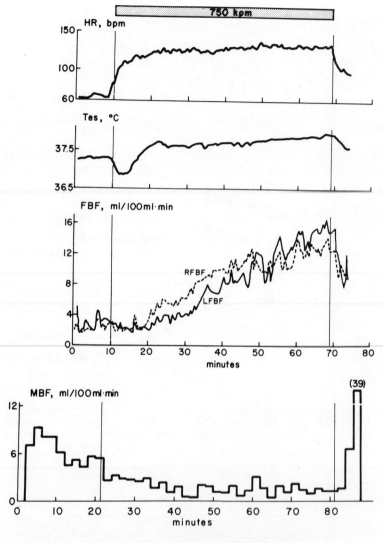

FIG. 9. *Response of total forearm blood flow in right and left arms (RFBF and LFBF) in one subject during 1 hr of exercise at 750 kpm/min at 24°C ambient. The bottom panel from a separate experiment shows that the increase in FBF was confined to skin. Forearm muscle blood flow (^{125}I-antipyrine clearance) fell during exercise. (From Johnson et al. [17], by permission of the American Physiological Society.)*

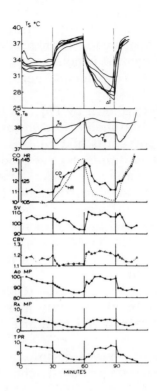

FIG. 10. Overall circulatory responses to rapid
changes in whole body skin temperature (T_s) during upright exercise. From top to bottom, panels
show the time course of T_s, rectal (T_r) and right
atrial blood temperature (T_{ra}), cardiac output
(CO,L/min) and heart rate (HR, bpm), stroke volume (SV, ml), central blood volume (CBV, liters),
aortic mean pressure (AoMP, mm Hg), right atrial
mean pressure (RaMP, mm Hg) and total peripheral
resistance (TPR, mm Hg/L·min). Note the fall in
SV, CBV, AoMP, and RaMP with each elevation in T_s
(30 and 90 min) and the sudden increase in these
variables when T_s was suddenly lowered at 60 min
(see text for details). (Modified from Rowell
et al. [34].)

T_S was held at 32 to 33°C and accelerated when T_s was raised toward 38°C at 30 min. Vasodilation in the skin, as predicted above, caused a sudden fall in central blood volume (CBV) (see Fig. 4) while the downward drift in central venous pressure and aortic mean pressure continued. Stroke volume fell during heating. Changes in central venous pressure and stroke volume were more obvious during the second period of heating after 90 min.

Another major finding shown by Fig. 10 is that cooling the skin for 60 to 90 min abolished all downward drift in stroke volume, aortic mean pressure, and central venous pressure. Thus, heating must have displaced the blood volume from the central vasculature to cutaneous veins, whereas cooling must have caused cutaneous venoconstriction. Note in Fig. 10 the sudden increases in central blood volume, stroke volume, central venous pressure and blood pressure when T_s was suddenly decreased. Referring again to Fig. 4, we can see that cooling caused venous return to the right heart to exceed momentarily the output of the left ventricle so that the volumes of pre-right and left ventricular sumps (CBV for the left ventricle) and filling pressures were rapidly increased. The opposite occurred when T_s was raised and skin arterioles (and veins, see below) were relaxed.

Changes in cutaneous venous compliance with heat stress during exercise may also contribute to the changes in central blood volume, pressures, etc. illustrated in Fig. 10. At normal skin and core temperatures, venous tone is very low in resting man; the effects of increasing T_s and T_c on venous compliance are therefore relatively small (20, 37). Upright exercise is attended, however, by reflex venoconstriction in the skin. Presumably, this response serves to reduce skin venous volume and thus minimize any transient lag in venous return from the skin at the onset of exercise.

Fig. 11 illustrates the effects of both direct local and reflex effects of heating on cutaneous venous tone. Venous tone was determined from changes in forearm venous pressure while both forearm arteries and veins were totally occluded (30, 31). The upper panel of Fig. 11 shows the rapid venoconstriction at the onset of exercise while body T_s was held at 34°C (neutral temperature). When local arm T_s was cycled between 32 and 40°C, the veins slowly relaxed on heating and constricted again with local cooling. In contrast, the bottom panel shows the rapid loss of venous tone when whole body T_s was increased

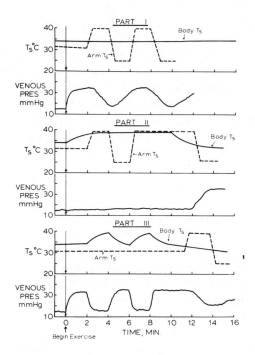

FIG. 11. *Changes in tone of forearm cutaneous veins during exercise in response to changes in local arm T_S and whole body T_S with arm T_S held at different temperatures. The veins constricted (rise in pressure within occluded veins) with the onset of exercise (arrow at time 0 min). The top panel (Part I) shows slow changes in venous tone with changes in local arm T_S. In contrast, there were rapid venomotor responses when body T_S was cycled (Part III, bottom panel). In Part II, center panel, note that local arm T_S had no effect on venous tone as long as body T_S was elevated. See text for explanation. (Modified from Rowell et al. [31].)*

toward 38°C; venous tone was rapidly restored when T_S began to fall. Arm T_S was held at 32°C during these cycles of whole body T_S. But when body T_S was raised to 38°C before exercise began (middle panel), no venoconstriction occurred with exercise and cycling of local arm T_S had no effect on venous tone. Taken together, these results reveal two separate effects of cutaneous heating (note that in these brief experiments changes in T_{ra} were in the wrong direction to explain the results[30, 31]). Raising body T_S reflexly decreased the rate of sympathetic nerve outflow to veins, so that even when arm veins were locally cooled, and thus maximally reactive to nerve stimulation, no venoconstriction occurred. Conversely, altering local arm T_S simply altered the reactivity of cutaneous veins to sympathetic nerve stimulation. When nerve stimulation was present (i.e., at low body T_S), the veins responded to local temperature changes. When there was no sympathetic nerve activity reaching the veins (i.e., at elevated body T_S), then local temperature changes were without effect. Webb-Peploe and Shepherd (41) observed similar phenomena in the cutaneous veins of the dog limb when T_C was altered. Just how skin and central temperatures interact to control cutaneous veins is an unsolved problem in temperature regulation.

The above observations reinforce a point made earlier; namely, any check on the volume of blood displaced to the skin during upright exercise must occur on the arterial side of the circulation through vasoconstriction. Through both local and reflex effects, increases in T_C and T_S will relax venous tone and favor a shift of blood volume into cutaneous veins. At any given skin blood flow, this volume shift favors heat loss by reducing the linear flow velocity directly beneath the skin.

Studies carried out in natural environments have yielded results similar to those generated by driving T_S with water-perfused suits (27, 43). The major difference is in the response of cardiac output; it increased 2 to 4 L/min when T_S is suddenly raised by water-perfused suits. Johnson et al. (manuscript in preparation) recently showed that much of the rise in skin blood flow in these suits is due to the direct local effects of heat on skin blood vessels. When responses of six men to exercise at an ambient temperature of 25°C were compared with their responses at 43°C, both stroke volume and central blood volume were decreased at all intensities of exercise that required 43 to 86 per cent of $\dot{V}_{O_2}$ max (Fig. 12) (33). At a given

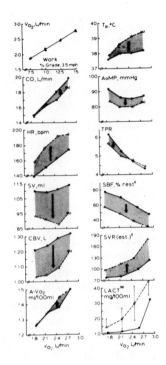

FIG. 12. Cardiovascular responses to graded exercise in hot (43.3°C Δ---Δ) and neutral
(25.6°C •——•) environments. The upper left-hand
panel shows $\dot{V}_{O_2}$ vs. work intensity to illustrate
absence of temperature effects on $\dot{V}_{O_2}$. All data
in remaining panels are plotted against $\dot{V}_{O_2}$ during
exercise. Arrows show the direction of tempera-
ture-induced change in each variable. Variables,
CO, HR, SV, CBV, T_r, AoMP, and TPR, are defined
in legend for Fig. 10. Other variables are
splanchnic blood flow (SBF, as per cent of the
resting value - 100%), estimated splanchnic vascular resistance (SVR) and blood lactate concentration (LACT). (From Rowell [27], by permission of the American Physiological Society.)

$\dot{V}_{O_2}$ at 43° C, cardiac output was maintained up to a point but not increased by augmented heart rate. As a result of reduced stroke volume, maximal heart rate (195 beats/min) was reached at 2.8 L O_2/min at 43° C rather than at 3.8 L O_2/min (the $\dot{V}_{O_2}$ max), as occurred at 25° C. If anything, heat stress at the higher intensities of exercise tended to lower cardiac output.

The findings summarized in Fig. 12 suggest that skin blood flow could not have increased much during exercise despite severe hyperthermia (T_c reached 40° C at the end of the highest rates of work). A study of identical design showed that splanchnic blood flow is further reduced at any given $\dot{V}_{O_2}$ by added heat stress (29). Also, the reduction in renal blood flow at any given $\dot{V}_{O_2}$ during exercise is augmented by heat stress (24). These major vascular beds could redistribute, however, only an additional 600 to 800 ml of blood per min to the skin. From the available data for total and regional blood flow (27, 40), some upper limits for skin blood flow during exercise have been estimated (27). The assumptions were that all blood flow redistributed from splanchnic and renal beds is directed to the skin along with that redistributed from resting and working skeletal muscle. The maximal contribution from working muscle was derived by calculation of the minimum muscle blood flow necessary to maintain $\dot{V}_{O_2}$ at each workload, on the assumption of 100 percent extraction of oxygen by the muscle (c.f., 27). It appears that skin blood flow could not exceed 3 to 4 L/min at low rates of work or 2 to 3 L/min at higher work intensities. There simply is not enough cardiac output or regional blood flow available to raise skin blood flow to the levels seen at rest at equivalent levels of T_c. This conclusion is directly supported by Johnson and colleagues' (18) observation of a much lower forearm skin blood flow at any given T_c during upright exercise than during supine rest. Further, man can reach his $\dot{V}_{O_2}$ max in hot environments when T_c is elevated (32). Clearly, the skin is vasoconstricted at $\dot{V}_{O_2}$ max, since any significant cutaneous vasodilation would lower $\dot{V}_{O_2}$ max; that is, most of the "maximal" cardiac output must be distributed to working muscle for $\dot{V}_{O_2}$ max to be achieved, as outlined previously (27). It should be noted, however, that severe heat stress can lower $\dot{V}_{O_2}$ max (36), once vasodilator drive to the skin can partially overcome cutaneous vasoconstriction.

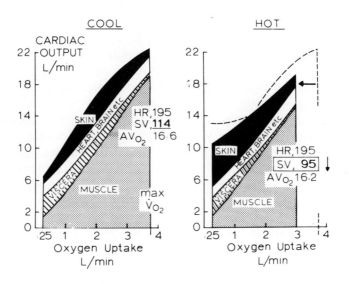

FIG. 13. *Estimated distribution of cardiac output in relation to oxygen uptake during upright exercise in neutral (25.6°C) and hot (43.3°C) environments. Data for CO vs. $\dot{V}O_2$ and values for HR, SV and A-VO_2 (symbols defined in legend for Fig. 10) were compiled from several investigations (see references 18, 24, 27-29, 33, 40). In hot environments, circulatory capacity may be reached at 3.0 rather than 3.7 L/min ($\dot{V}O_2$ max at 25.6°C) owing to reduction in SV (from 114 to 95 [33]) and attainment of maximal HR (195 bpm) at submaximal $\dot{V}O_2$. Thus, in contrast to the scheme illustrated in Fig. 1, $\dot{V}O_2$ max may be reduced under severe heat stress, not because skin blood flow is so high, but because the reduction in SV results in reduced maximal CO. (Note that although this state appears to be reached during progressive hyperthermia, some subjects can still elicit sufficient vasoconstrictor drive for brief periods to permit attainment of true $\dot{V}O_2$ max [32]). (From Rowell [27], by permission of the American Physiological Society.)*

The general concept that emerges is that upright posture and exercise cause a generalized increase in sympathetic nervous outflow. The outflow is further augmented when heat stress is superimposed upon exercise. The recipients of this increased vasoconstrictor activity include renal, splanchnic and cutaneous vascular beds. This pattern of sympathetic nervous activity not only optimizes the distribution of cardiac output but also checks peripheral displacement of blood volume. Thus, reductions in central blood volume, stroke volume, and blood pressure are minimized. Recent evidence, therefore, reveals that the hypothesis illustrated in Fig. 1 is indeed incorrect. Fig. 13 summarizes some current findings and estimates the distribution of cardiac output to skin and other regions during combined exercise and heat stress. The major difference from Brouha's scheme is that skin blood flow and cardiac output do not show the marked increases postulated by some.

The title of this symposium refers to "problems in temperature regulation, " but the problems are seen with varying perspective in this broad interdisciplinary field. The cardiovascular physiologist sees temperature regulation as principally a cardiovascular problem, and this chapter focuses upon problems in regulation of blood pressure, total and regional blood flow, and blood volume distribution during heat stress and exercise. A clear understanding of some of the key problems in temperature regulation awaits solution of some major experimental problems. The following are a few examples:

i) As yet, we have no adequate measurement of total skin blood flow during exercise. Crude estimates of "skin conductance" or "thermal circulation index" have not been helpful for reasons outlined by Brown and Brengelmann (6), for example. It would be helpful to know whether the working skeletal muscle is a target of increased sympathetic nervous activity during exercise and heat stress. Donald et al. (9) demonstrated in dogs that the working skeletal muscle will vasoconstrict when its sympathetic nerve supply is directly stimulated. Were this to occur reflexly in man at submaximal exercise, then substantial quantities of blood flow could be redistributed from the working muscle to the skin. In fact, this appears to be the only way skin blood flow could reach levels greater than those postulated in Fig. 13. A solution awaits better methods of measuring blood flow to active muscle in man.

ii) Ninety to 100 per cent of the increase in skin blood flow (depending on the baseline level of vasoconstrictor tone to skin) in hyperthermic man is due to increased activity of a neurogenic, active vasodilator system (14, 26, 28, 37). Cutaneous vasodilation has been linked to sweating and local bradykinin formation (12), but evidence has been challenged (c.f., 28). In short, we still do not understand how the skin vasodilates. This potent vasodilator system is the major arm of temperature regulation in hyperthermic man. As far as we know it is unique; it is even absent in subhuman primates who show thermal sweating (46). The great capacities of both this dilator system and thermal sweating in man explain his remarkable thermoregulatory ability.

iii) We do not yet understand the relative roles of T_s and T_c in the control of skin blood flow during exercise. When man is at rest in a neutral environment and tonic vasoconstrictor outflow to the skin is relatively minor, a 1°C rise in body T_s exerts only about one twentieth of the effect on skin blood flow as a 1°C rise in T_c (44, 45). Available evidence suggests that the changes in T_s act primarily on vasoconstrictor activity to the skin, whereas the changes in T_c activate the vasodilator system. During exercise, however, as vasoconstrictor outflow to the skin is increased and it competes with vasodilator outflow, any release of tonic vasoconstrictor activity to the skin by a rise of body T_s should have a marked effect on skin blood flow. This response is suggested by the dramatic effects of increased T_s on cardiac output, heart rate, etc. during upright exercise shown in Fig. 10. Note that these changes were coincident with a fall in T_{ra}.

Clearly, since some of these experimental problems are unique to man, they can only be solved with human subjects. Solutions await adequate pharmacological means of separating the vasoconstrictor and vasodilator effector mechanisms in the skin.

Directly associated with the experimental problems outlined above are some conceptual problems. A major point in this chapter is that thermoregulatory control of the skin circulation cannot be considered separate from other reflex inputs. For example, Fig. 14 illustrates a more traditional view of the control of the cutaneous circulation. In this scheme, reflex control is mediated via drives from cutaneous and central thermoreceptors. The efferent arm in man involves the vasoconstrictor and vasodilator effector mechanisms discussed above, but this scheme provides no basis for understanding the nature of the competition between skin and muscle blood

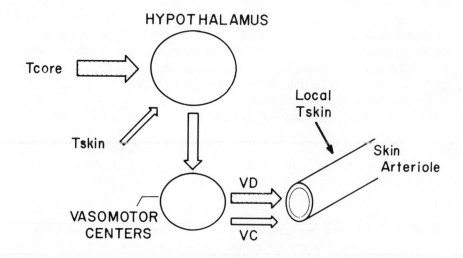

FIG. 14. A traditional scheme of human cutaneous
vascular control. Cutaneous thermoreceptors
respond to changes in skin temperature (T_{skin}),
and central thermoreceptors (hypothalamus)
respond to changes in skin and core temperature
(T_{core}). Reflex control of skin arterioles is
modulated via sympathetic vasodilator (VD) and
sympathetic vasoconstrictor (VC) nervous out-
flows from vasomotor centers. The VD drive is
the major component in thermoregulatory control
of skin blood flow and body temperature (with
adequate evaporation of sweat) in heat-stressed
man.

flow during exercise, for example. In Fig. 15, a revised
scheme illustrates the basis for this competition by placing
other major inputs to vasomotor "centers" within the regulatory framework. A goal of this chapter is to illustrate that
even during heat stress, skin can fall under the dominant
influence of the sympathetic vasoconstrictor drive emanating
from vasomotor "centers". The skin is on the efferent side of

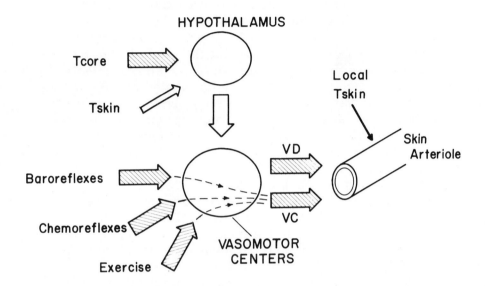

FIG. 15. *A scheme illustrating some major factors contributing to regulation of skin blood
flow in man. This scheme adds to those in Fig.
14 other major inputs acting on skin arterioles
via sympathetic vasoconstrictor (VC) nerves.
These nonthermoregulatory inputs are thought to
act only through modulation of VC outflow
(dashed lines); they can be major determinants of
skin blood flow even during heat stress when vasodilator (VD) drive is also augmented.*

reflexes elicited by (i) falling arterial blood pressure, mediated
by arterial baroreceptors (4, 35); (ii) falling central venous
pressure, mediated via cardiopulmonary baroreceptors (19)
(note that central venous pressure decreases in upright man
during heat stress); and by (iii) supine or upright exercise (18).
When stresses are severe, temperature regulation can give way
to blood pressure regulation, or vice versa.

Unfortunately, we do not know where the integration of vasoconstrictor and vasodilator drives takes place. Does vasoconstrictor outflow compete with vasodilator outflow merely at receptor sites on cutaneous resistance vessels? Conversely, is there feedback so that vasodilator outflow is also centrally modulated by nonthermoregulatory reflexes? Again, we must find a way to separate these two effector mechanisms in man. It may turn out that a change in the so-called thermoregulatory set-point during exercise reflects nothing more than the effects of an augmented background bias of sympathetic vasoconstrictor activity during exercise. This vasoconstrictor bias changes the intercept and possibly the slope of the skin blood flow– T_c relationship (18); the result of a relatively vasoconstricted skin is an elevated T_c as body heat elimination is reduced.

The thermoregulation-physiologists' view of the skin circulation appears to have been narrow when viewed in the perspective of cardiovascular physiology. To view skin blood flow as the sole province of temperature regulation and ignore the consequences for overall cardiovascular regulation is clearly not valid. The skin, even during heat stress, can be as much a target of reflex vasoconstrictor activity as other major vascular regions; indeed this condition must exist if heat-stressed man is to remain upright without syncope.

References

1.   Amberson, W. R. Physiologic adjustments to the standing posture. Bull. Maryland Univ. School Med. 27: 127-145, 1943.

2.   Asmussen, E. The distribution of the blood between the lower extremities and the rest of the body. Acta Physiol. Scand. 5: 31-38, 1943.

3.   Barcroft, H., K. D. Bock, H. Hensel, and A.H. Kitchin. Die Muskeldurchblutung des Menschen bei indirekter Erwärmung und Abkühlung. Arch. Ges. Physiol. 261: 199-210, 1955.

4.   Beiser, G. D., R. Zelis, S. E. Epstein, D. T. Mason, and E. Braunwald. The role of skin and muscle resistance vessels in reflexes mediated by the baroreceptor system. J. Clin. Invest. 49: 225-231, 1970.

5.   Brouha, L. Physiologic effect of work on the heart.
In: The Heart in Industry, edited by L. J. Warshaw.
New York: Paul B. Hoeber, Inc., 1960, chapt. 2,
p. 47-104.

6.   Brown, A. C., and G. L. Brengelmann. The interaction
of peripheral and central inputs in the temperature regulation system. In: Physiological and Behavioral Temperature Regulation, edited by J. D. Hardy, A.P. Gagge,
and J. A. J. Stolwijk. Springfield, Ill.: Charles C.
Thomas, 1970, chapt. 47, p. 684-702.

7.   Crossley, R. J., A. D. M. Greenfield, G. C. Plassaras,
and D. Stephens. The interrelation of thermoregulatory
and baroreceptor reflexes in the control of the blood
vessels in the human forearm. J. Physiol., London
183: 628-636, 1966.

8.   Detry, J.-M. R., G. L. Brengelmann, L. B. Rowell,
and C. Wyss. Skin and muscle components of forearm
blood flow in directly heated resting man. J. Appl.
Physiol. 32: 506-511, 1972.

9.   Donald, D. E., D. J. Rowlands, and D. A. Ferguson.
Similarity of blood flow in the normal and the sympathec-
tomized dog hind limb during graded exercise. Circulation Res. 26: 185-199, 1970.

10.   Edholm, O. G., R. H. Fox, and R. K. MacPherson.
The effect of body heating on the circulation in skin
and muscle. J. Physiol., London 134: 612-619, 1956.

11.   Ekelund, L.-G. Circulatory and respiratory adaptation
during prolonged exercise. Acta Physiol. Scand. 70,
Suppl. 292: 1967.

12.   Fox, R. H., and S. M. Hilton. Bradykinin formation
in human skin as a factor in heat vasodilatation. J.
Physiol., London 142: 219-232, 1958.

13.   Gauer, O. H., and H. L. Thron. Postural changes in
the circulation. In: Handbook of Physiology, Circulation, edited by W. F. Hamilton and P. Dow. Washington, D. C.: American Physiological Society, 1965,
sect. 2, vol. III, chapt. 67, p. 2409-2439.

14.   Greenfield, A. D. M. The circulation through the skin.
In: Handbook of Physiology, Circulation, edited by
W. F. Hamilton and P. Dow. Washington, D. C.:
American Physiological Society, 1963, sect. 2, vol. II,
chapt. 39, p. 1325-1351.

15. Henry, J. P., and O. H. Gauer. The influence of temperature upon venous pressure in the foot. J. Clin. Invest. 29: 855-861, 1950.

16. Johnson, J. M., M. Niederberger, L. B. Rowell, M. M. Eisman, and G. L. Brengelmann. Competition between cutaneous vasodilator and vasoconstrictor reflexes in man. J. Appl. Physiol. 35: 798-803, 1973.

17. Johnson, J. M., and L. B. Rowell. Forearm skin and muscle vascular responses to prolonged leg exercise in man. J. Appl. Physiol. 39: 920-924, 1975.

18. Johnson, J. M., L. B. Rowell, and G. L. Brengelmann. Modification of the skin blood flow–body temperature relationship by upright exercise. J. Appl. Physiol. 37: 880-886, 1974.

19. Johnson, J. M., L. B. Rowell, M. Niederberger, and M. M. Eisman. Human splanchnic and forearm vasoconstrictor responses to reductions of right atrial and aortic pressures. Circulation Res. 34:515-524, 1974.

20. Kidd, B. S. L., and S. M. Lyons. The distensibility of the blood vessels of the human calf determined by graded venous congestion. J. Physiol., London, 140: 122-128, 1958.

21. Lind, A. R., C. S. Leithead, and G. W. McNicol. Cardiovascular changes during syncope induced by tilting men in the heat. J. Appl. Physiol. 25: 268-276, 1968.

22. Mosley, J. G. A. A reduction in some vasodilator responses in freestanding man. Cardiovascular Res. 3: 14-21, 1969.

23. Nielsen, M., L. P. Herrington, and C.-E. A. Winslow. The effect of posture on peripheral circulation. Am. J. Physiol. 127: 573-580, 1939.

24. Radigan, L. R., and S. Robinson. Effects of environmental heat stress and exercise on renal blood flow and filtration rate. J. Appl. Physiol. 2:185-191, 1949.

25. Roddie, I. C., J. T. Shepherd, and R. F. Whelan. Evidence from venous oxygen saturation measurements that the increase in forearm blood flow during body heating is confined to the skin. J. Physiol., London 134: 444-450, 1956.

26. Roddie, I. C., J. T. Shepherd, and R. F. Whelan. The contribution of constrictor and dilator nerves to the skin vasodilatation during body heating. *J. Physiol.*, *London* 136: 489-497, 1957.

27. Rowell, L. B. Human cardiovascular adjustments to exercise and thermal stress. *Physiol. Rev.* 54: 75-159, 1974.

28. Rowell, L. B. The Cutaneous Circulation. In: *Textbook of Physiology and Biophysics*, edited by T. C. Ruch and H. D. Patton. Philadelphia: Saunders, 1974, 20th ed., vol. II, chapt. 12, p. 185-199.

29. Rowell, L. B., J. R. Blackmon, R. H. Martin, J. A. Mazzarella, and R. A. Bruce. Hepatic clearance of indocyanine green in man under thermal and exercise stresses. *J. Appl. Physiol.* 20: 384-394, 1965.

30. Rowell, L. B., G. L. Brengelmann, J.-M.R. Detry, and C. Wyss. Venomotor responses to rapid changes in skin temperature in exercising man. *J. Appl. Physiol.* 30: 64-71, 1971.

31. Rowell, L. B., G. L. Brengelmann, J.-M. R. Detry, and C. Wyss. Venomotor responses to local and remote thermal stimuli to skin in exercising man. *J. Appl. Physiol.* 30: 72-77, 1971.

32. Rowell, L. B., G. L. Brengelmann, J. A. Murray, K. K. Kraning, II, and F. Kusumi. Human metabolic responses to hyperthermia during mild to maximal exercise. *J. Appl. Physiol.* 26: 395-402, 1969.

33. Rowell, L. B., H. J. Marx, R. A. Bruce, R. D. Conn, and F. Kusumi. Reductions in cardiac output, central blood volume, and stroke volume with thermal stress in normal men during exercise. *J. Clin. Invest.* 45: 1801-1816, 1966.

34. Rowell, L. B., J. A. Murray, G. L. Brengelmann, and K. K. Kraning. Human cardiovascular adjustments to rapid changes in skin temperature. *Circulation Res.* 24: 711-724, 1969.

35. Rowell, L. B., C. R. Wyss, and G. L. Brengelmann. Sustained human skin and muscle vasoconstriction with reduced baroreceptor activity. *J. Appl. Physiol.* 34: 639-643, 1973.

36. Saltin, B., A. P. Gagge, U. Bergh, and J.A.J. Stolwijk. Body temperatures and sweating during exhaustive exercise. *J. Appl. Physiol.* 32: 635-643, 1972.

37. Shepherd, J. T. Physiology of the Circulation in Human Limbs in Health and Disease. Philadelphia: Saunders, 1963.
38. Shepherd, J. T. Role of the veins in the circulation. Circulation 33: 484-491, 1966.
39. Shepherd, J. T., and P. M. Vanhoutte. Veins and Their Control. London: Saunders, 1975, chapt. 2, p. 21-51.
40. Wade, O. L., and J. M. Bishop. Cardiac Output and Regional Blood Flow. Oxford: Blackwell, 1962.
41. Webb-Peploe, M. M., and J. T. Shepherd. Responses of dogs' cutaneous veins to local and central temperature changes. Circulation Res. 23: 693-699, 1968.
42. Webb-Peploe, M. M., and J. T. Shepherd. Veins and their control. New Eng. J. Med. 278: 317-322, 1968.
43. Wyndham, C. H. The physiology of exercise under heat stress. Ann. Rev. Physiol. 35: 193-220, 1973.
44. Wyss, C. R., G. L. Brengelmann, J. M. Johnson, L. B. Rowell, and M. Niederberger. Control of skin blood flow, sweating and heart rate: role of skin vs. core temperature. J. Appl. Physiol. 36: 726-733, 1974.
45. Wyss, C. R., G. L. Brengelmann, J. M. Johnson, L. B. Rowell, and D. Silverstein. Altered control of skin blood flow at high skin and core temperatures. J. Appl. Physiol. 38: 839-845, 1975.
46. Wyss, C. R., and L. B. Rowell. Lack of human-like active vasodilation in skin of heat-stressed baboons. J. Appl. Physiol., in press, 1976.

Changes in Thermoregulatory and Cardiovascular Function with Heat Acclimation

Jan A. J. Stolwijk, Michael F. Roberts
C. Bruce Wenger, and Ethan R. Nadel

Challenges to the thermoregulatory system arise in situations which bring about an increase in body (i.e., core and skin) temperatures. As body temperatures rise, proportional increases in two important physiological responses cause an increase in heat loss: vasodilation in the skin increases the thermal conductance between body core and skin, and sweating transfers heat to the environment by evaporation from the skin surface. Thus, any thermal stress due to hot environment or physical activity will cause a rise in body temperature until the elevated temperatures bring avenues of heat loss into play which are equivalent to the levels of heat gain from environment or activity.

If the stress exceeds the capability of the thermoregulatory heat loss mechanisms, the core temperature will continue to rise until heat stroke ultimately occurs (19). In addition, lesser degrees of heat stress, which are within the capacity of the thermoregulatory system, may produce heat strain in the form of such heat disorders as syncope and heat exhaustion. A milder form of heat strain, but one which is important and has often been studied in the laboratory is manifested in high heart rate, high body temperatures, and inability to perform prolonged heavy exercise in the heat. If persons who show this type of strain on an initial heat exposure continue to exercise in a hot environment for a number of days, they show an increased sweat rate, and striking reductions in heart rate and body temperatures, as well as improved ability to exercise in the heat (14, 25).

The improved exercise tolerance probably owes to reduced heart rate and increased cardiac stroke volume. Rowell et al. (15) attributed the decrease in heart rate to the reduced body temperatures which accompany acclimation, and they considered that the increase in stroke volume occurs secondarily to the lower heart rate. Senay et al. (17, 18) and Wyndham et al. (26) postulated that stroke volume increases through an acclimation-induced increase in plasma volume, and that the lower heart rate is allowed by this increase in stroke volume. Increased plasma volume has been reported in several studies (2, 16, 18, 26). One acclimation study, by Bass et al. (1) showed no change in plasma volume, but this study employed a comparatively mild thermal stress. Another factor contributing to increased stroke volume may be increased venomotor tone (23, 24), which would be expected to act in the same manner as increased plasma volume to increase filling pressure. Unfortunately, no measurements of filling pressure have been made in studies of heat acclimation (14), so the mechanism for the changes in heart rate and stroke volume remains uncertain.

A feature of experimental design which complicates comparison between studies is the use of dry vs. humid heat during acclimation. Eichna et al. (3) and Rowell et al. (15), using dry heat, reported that core to skin thermal gradient widened over a ten day exposure period, implying a decrease in skin blood flow. Mitchell et al. (7), using humid heat, showed no change in thermal gradient of the subjects in their study, even though both core and skin temperatures fell over the exposure period. In this study, it is likely that the low evaporating power of the humid environment limited the fall in T_{sk}. Since core temperature also declined somewhat, a widening of the core to skin thermal gradient may thus have been prevented.

A number of investigators (5, 11, 12) have reported that highly trained subjects exhibited many of the characteristics of heat-acclimated individuals during exercise in the heat. Other investigators (20) have found that training resulted in partial acclimation, but maintained that physical training in a cool environment was not able to provide complete acclimation to exercise in a hot environment, since heat tolerance of trained subjects was increased further by heat acclimation. Thus, factors associated with exercise training may be important in the total heat acclimation response, but as Wyndham has recently noted (25), these do not account for the entire response.

Consistent with this, we have recently reported (10) that exercise training increased the slope of the sweat rate: internal temperature relation, and heat acclimation shifted the internal temperature threshold for sweating toward lower internal temperatures. Thus training increases sweating at a

given internal temperature, to allow the heat produced during
exercise to be dissipated at lower body temperatures than before training, and acclimation further augments this effect.

In the study to be described, we were interested in the
changes which may occur in the relation of skin blood flow
to internal temperature, as a result of a similar program of
exercise training and heat acclimation.

Characterization of thermoregulatory responses. To determine
how the thermoregulatory control of sweating and skin blood
flow changes with exercise training and heat acclimation, we
determined the relations of sweating and of forearm blood flow
to internal temperature, before and after successive programs
of exercise training and heat acclimation.

Blood flow in the forearm (ABF) was measured by electro-
capacitance plethysmograph (21), and sweating $(\dot{m}_{sw})$ was
measured by resistance hygrometry from a 13 cm^2 capsule on
the chest (8). Internal temperature (T_{es}) was measured in
the esophagus at the level of the left atrium, and mean skin
temperature $(\bar{T}_{sk})$ was computed from a weighted mean of three
skin temperature measurements (chest, lateral thigh, and
lateral upper arm). We have previously shown (9, 21) that the
effect on sweating and blood flow of a change in T_{es} is about
10 times that of the same change in $\bar{T}_{sk}$.

A representative experiment for determining the $\dot{m}_{sw}$:T_{es}
and ABF:T_{es} relations is shown in Fig. 1. At the onset of
exercise, T_{es} decreased slightly, then rose continuously
during exercise. As T_{es} increased above 37.3° C, sweating
began and rose proportionally with T_{es}. Similarly, ABF increased proportionally with T_{es} above 37.5° C. Mean skin
temperature declined slightly during the exercise period.

Figure 2 illustrates the $\dot{m}_{sw}$:T_{es} and ABF:T_{es} relations
obtained from Fig. 1. Both relations are linear with T_{es} above
their threshold values and illustrate the control of these heat
dissipation responses in an unacclimated, untrained subject.

Effect of exercise training and heat acclimation on thermoregulatory response. The initial maximum aerobic power
$(\dot{V}O_2$ max) was determined in an incremental exercise test on
a bicycle ergometer, and thresholds and slopes of the
$\dot{m}_{sw}$:T_{es} and ABF:T_{es} relations were determined in duplicate
tests on separate days at an ambient temperature of 25° C.

Exercise training was then accomplished by having the subjects exercise on a bicycle ergometer for one hour per day (four 15 min exercise periods separated by 5 min rest periods) on ten consecutive days at an ambient temperature of 23-25°C. The exercise intensity was adjusted so that the heart rate was maintained between 160 and 170 beats per minute, representing a load of 78-80% $\dot{V}O_2$ max. At the end of the 10 days, $\dot{V}O_2$ max was determined again, as well as the thresholds and slopes of the sweating and forearm blood flow responses. The heat acclimation procedure began on the first day after the post-training tests. Subjects exercised at 50% $\dot{V}O_2$ max.

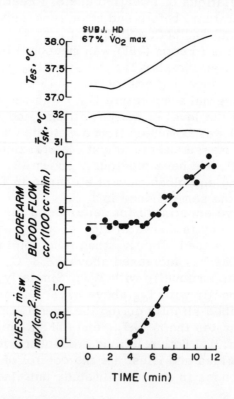

FIG. 1. *Time course of a typical experiment at an ambient temperature of 25°C showing (from top) esophageal temperature, mean skin temperature, forearm blood flow, and sweating rate on the chest. (From Roberts et al. (13), with permission of American Physiological Society.)*

for 10 consecutive days for 1 hour per day (two 30 min exercise periods separated by a 15 min rest period) in either a hot-dry (45°C, 16 Torr water vapor pressure) or a warm-humid (35°C, 35 Torr water vapor pressure) environment. Heart rate was measured each day during the final minute of exercise, and rectal temperature was measured immediately after the end of exercise. At the end of this acclimation period, the final tests of $\dot{V}O_2$ max and of the characteristics of sweating and forearm blood flow responses were made. As Fig. 3 shows, exercise training produced a substantial increase in $\dot{V}O_2$ max. Subsequent exercise in the heat for 10 days did not produce any consistent further increase in $\dot{V}O_2$ max. Figure 3 also shows the substantial reductions in heart rate and core temperature during the same 10 day period of heat acclimation.

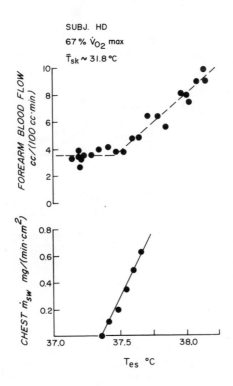

FIG. 2.   Data from Fig. 1 replotted to show linear relation of forearm blood flow and sweat rate to esophageal temperature.

These results demonstrate the beneficial effects of heat acclimation: lowered core temperature and lowered heart rate for a given work load in the heat.

Effect of training and acclimation on the thermoregulatory system.   These changes are accompanied by quantitative changes in the control of the sweating and vasodilation responses, as indicated in Figures 4 and 5.

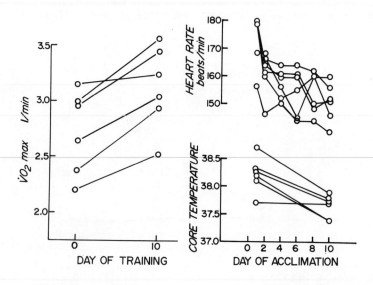

FIG. 3. (left). *Maximum aerobic power of six subjects before and after 10 days of exercise training. (Right.) Heart rates and rectal temperatures of the same six subjects during the subsequent program of heat acclimation. (From Nadel et al. (10), with permission of the American Physiological Society).*

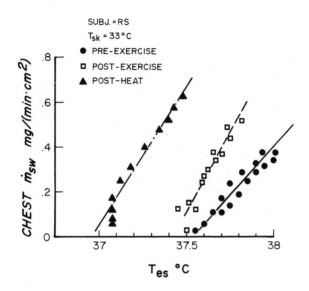

FIG. 4. Chest sweating rate plotted against esophageal temperature of a subject exercising in an ambient temperature of 25°C. Circles = pre-training data; squares = post training data; triangles = post heat acclimation data. (From Roberts et al. (13), with permission of American Physiological Society).

In our test conditions at 25°C ambient temperature, $\bar{T}_{sk}$ showed only small and inconsistent changes with training and acclimation, and thus cannot account for the changes in the ABF:T_{es} and $\dot{m}_{sw}$:T_{es} relations. Although subjects do not all show exactly the same changes, the general trend is that exercise training increases the slope of the sweating response, with only a slight reduction in the T_{es} threshold for sweating (Fig. 4). It is seen in Fig. 5 that in this subject the forearm blood flow response is essentially unaffected by

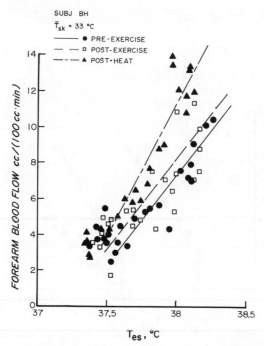

FIG. 5. *Forearm blood flow plotted against esophageal temperature of a subject exercising at an ambient temperature of 25°C. Circles = pretraining data; squares = post training data; triangles = post heat acclimation data (From Roberts et al. (13), with permission of American Physiological Society).*

exercise training, except for a small shift toward lower values of T_{es}. To the extent that cardiovascular strain limits the ability to work in the heat, exercise training improves the overall tolerance to such conditions and the capability to perform such work. For a given set of conditions, the sweat rate required for thermal equilibrium is reached at a lower body temperature, and since the forearm blood flow response is essentially unchanged, this will mean that the same work load is performed with a lower cardiovascular demand.

Figures 4 and 5 also show the changes in thermoregulatory response following heat acclimation. Both sweating and blood flow maintain approximately the same slope, but the thresholds are lowered by about $0.3°C$. This would clearly result in a lowered body temperature during exercise at a given intensity and ambient temperature, but it is not evident here how the clear benefit of reduced heart rate is obtained, nor how the reduced core-to-skin thermal conductance observed after acclimation by a number of investigators (3, 15) is accomplished. These latter two changes suggest a lower value of peripheral blood flow at steady state during exercise in the heat. Since steady-state sweating rate is determined largely by the heat load to be dissipated, this implies that the relation between blood flow and sweating is changed toward lower levels of blood flow at any level of sweating. However, the threshold shifts in Figs. 4 and 5 do not explain such a change. In fact, similar shifts in thresholds are observed as a function of the time of day (22), as shown in Fig. 6; if these threshold shifts were of importance to tolerance for work in the heat, then there should be a considerable improvement in tolerance to work in the heat during the early morning. We are now aware of reports of greatly improved tolerance to work in the heat in the early morning hours.

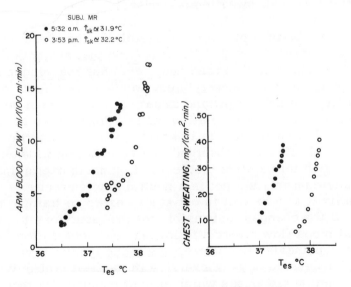

FIG. 6. The relations of chest sweating and of forearm blood flow to esophageal temperature during exercise in the early morning (filled circles) and in the afternoon (open circles). (From Wenger et al. (22), with permission of American Physiological Society.)

86   JAN A. J. STOLWIJK *et al.*

Beneficial effects of acclimation. Since the data in Figs. 4 and 5 do not account for the beneficial effects of acclimation, other explanations should be considered. These explanations, in turn, imply certain hypotheses, which may be tested more directly in future studies.

Fox et al. (4) have suggested that heat acclimation reduces the hidromeiotic effect, whereby a wet skin suppresses further sweat secretion locally. However, the skin under our sweat capsules was kept fairly dry by a current of air drawn through the capsule. Thus, our technique would fail to detect any effect of acclimation on hidromeiosis.

Hofler reported that most of the sweating of unacclimated subjects occurs on the trunk, but that the limbs provide most of the increase in sweating which accompanies heat acclimation (6). It is thus possible that in our acclimation study the sensitivity (i.e., slope with respect to T_{es}) of the chest sweating response was maximized by exercise training; but that other regions, which initially sweated less than the chest, continued during heat acclimation to increase the sensitivity of their sweating responses.

Furthermore, it should be noted that the data in Figs. 4 and 5 were obtained on subjects exercising for 15 min at an ambient temperature of 25° C. It may be that subjects exercising for long periods in the heat, and thus reaching much higher skin and core temperatures, would show effects of acclimation on blood flow and sweating which cannot be inferred from simply extrapolating the relations shown in Figs. 4 and 5. This suggestion is in keeping with the report of Eichna et al. (3), who observed that acclimation widened the core-to-skin temperature gradients of subjects exercising in a hot environment, but not in a neutral environment.

Finally it may be that in our study, exercise training alone produced the changes responsible for the reductions in peripheral blood flow reported following heat acclimation (3, 15). By this hypothesis, the progressive reductions in heart rate during successive days of exercise in the heat probably owe to acclimation responses which are not specifically thermoregulatory, but which improve circulatory function under conditions of heat stress.

Indeed, it is likely that such non-thermoregulatory responses participate in heat acclimation whatever the truth of the hypotheses set forth above. At a given level of cardiac output, heart rate is determined by cardiac stroke volume which, in turn depends to a large extent on cardiac filling pressure. Thus, any response which expands blood volume is likely to reduce heart rates during exercise in the heat. In a recent study of subjects who were being acclimated by working in a hot, humid environment, Senay et al. (18) obtained repeated measurements of heart rate and cardiac output, and estimated plasma volume changes from hemotocrits. Over the course of the acclimation program, they observed marked increases in initial resting plasma volume, which correlated strongly with increases in stroke volume and cardiac output, and with decreases in heart rate. Since their subjects showed no signs of change in core-to-skin temperature gradient over the course of acclimation (7), their plasma volume expansion seems to have been chiefly responsible for the cardiovascular improvements which they experienced. In their study, however, ambient water vapor pressure was so high that mean skin temperatures greater than 36° C were necessary to evaporate enough sweat to achieve thermal balance (7). For this reason, their results have uncertain application to acclimation in a hot dry environment.

Finally, Whitney (23) has suggested that a decrease in peripheral venous volume may accompany acclimation. In his study, this decrease seemed to occur in the absence of any reduction in peripheral blood flow. Such a change would probably contribute to cardiovascular improvements in the same manner as would expansion of plasma volume.

References

1. Bass, D. E., E. R. Buskirk, P. F. Iampietro, and M. Mager. Comparison of blood volume during physical conditioning, heat acclimatization and sedentary living. J. Appl. Physiol. 12: 186-188, 1958.
2. Bass, D. E., C. E. Kleeman, M. Quinn, A. Henschel, and A. H. Hegnauer. Mechanisms of acclimatization to heat. Medicine 34: 323-380, 1955.
3. Eichna, L. W., C. R. Park, N. Nelson, S. M. Horvath, and E. D. Palmes. Thermal regulation during acclimatization in hot, dry (desert type) environment. Am. J. Physiol. 163: 585-597, 1950.

4. Fox, R. H., B. E. Lofstedt, P. M. Woodward, E. Eriksson, and B. Werkstrom. Comparison of thermoregulatory function in men and women. J. Appl. Physiol. 26: 444-453, 1969.

5. Gisolfi, C., and S. Robinson. Relation between physical training, acclimatization, and heat tolerance. J. Appl. Physiol. 26: 530-534, 1969.

6. Hofler, W. Changes in regional distribution of sweating during acclimatization to heat. J. Appl. Physiol. 25: 503-506, 1968.

7. Mitchell, D., L. C. Senay, C. H. Wyndham, A. J. van Rensburg, G. G. Rogers, and N. B. Strydom. Acclimatization in a hot, humid environment: energy exchange, body temperature, and sweating. J. Appl. Physiol. 40: 768-778, 1976.

8. Nadel, E. R., R. W. Bullard, and J. A. J. Stolwijk. Importance of skin temperature in the regulation of sweating. J. Appl. Physiol. 31: 80-87, 1971.

9. Nadel, E. R., J. W. Mitchell, and J. A. J. Stolwijk. Control of local and total sweating during exercise transients. Intern. J. Biometeorol. 15: 201-206, 1971.

10. Nadel, E. R., K. B. Pandolf, M. F. Roberts, and J. A. J. Stolwijk. Mechanisms of thermal acclimation to exercise and heat. J. Appl. Physiol. 37: 515-520, 1974.

11. Piwonka, R. W., and S. Robinson. Acclimatization of highly trained men to work in severe heat. J. Appl. Physiol. 22: 9-12, 1967.

12. Piwonka, R. W., S. Robinson, V. L. Gay, and R. S. Manalis. Preacclimatization of men to heat by training. J. Appl. Physiol. 20: 379-384, 1965.

13. Roberts, M. F., C. B. Wenger, J. A. J. Stolwijk, and E. R. Nadel. Skin blood flow and sweating changes following exercise training and heat acclimation. J. Appl. Physiol. In press.

14. Rowell, L. B. Human cardiovascular adjustments to exercise and thermal stress. Physiol. Rev. 54: 75-159, 1974.

15. Rowell, L. B., K. K. Kraning, II, J. W. Kennedy, and T. O. Evans. Central circulatory responses to work in dry heat before and after acclimatization. J. Appl. Physiol. 22: 509-518, 1967.

16. Senay, L. C., Jr. Changes in plasma volume and protein content during exposures of working men to various temperatures before and after acclimatization to heat: separation of the roles of cutaneous and skeletal muscle circulation. J. Physiol., London 224: 61-81, 1972.

17. Senay, L. C., Jr. Plasma volumes and constituents of heat exposed men before and after acclimatization. J. Appl. Physiol. 38: 570-575, 1975.

18. Senay, L. C., Jr., D. Mitchell,and C. H. Wyndham. Acclimatization in a hot, humid environment: body fluid adjustments. J. Appl. Physiol. 40: 786-796, 1976.

19. Shibolet, S., M. C. Lancaster, and Y. Danon. Heat Stroke: a review. Aviat. Space Environ. Med. 47: 280-301, 1976.

20. Strydom, N. B., C. H Wyndham, C. G. Williams, J. F. Morrison, G. A. G. Bredell, A. J. S. Benade, and M. von Rahden. Acclimatization to humid heat and the role of physical conditioning. J. Appl. Physiol. 21: 636-642, 1966.

21. Wenger, C. B., M. F. Roberts, J. A. J. Stolwijk, and E. R. Nadel. Forearm blood flow during body temperature transients produced by leg exercise. J. Appl. Physiol. 38: 58-63, 1975.

22. Wenger, C. B., M. F. Roberts, J. A. J. Stolwijk, and E. R. Nadel. Nocturnal lowering of thresholds for sweating and vasodilation. J. Appl. Physiol. 41: 15-19, 1976.

23. Whitney, R. J. Circulatory changes in the forearm and hand of man with repeated exposure to heat. J. Physiol., London. 125: 1-24, 1954.

24. Wood, J. E., and D. E. Bass. Responses of the veins and arterioles of the forearm to walking during acclimatization to heat in man. J. Clin. Invest. 39: 825-833, 1960.

25. Wyndham, C. H. The physiology of exercise under heat stress. Ann. Rev. Physiol. 35: 193-220, 1973.

26. Wyndham, C. H., A. J. A. Benade, C. G. Williams, N. B. Strydom, A. Goldin, and A. J. A. Heyns. Changes in central circulation and body fluid spaces during acclimatization to heat. J. Appl. Physiol. 25: 586-593, 1968.

Acknowledgements

This study was partially supported by National Institutes of Health Grants ES-00123 and ES-00354, and by National Aeronautics and Space Administration Grant NSG-9023.

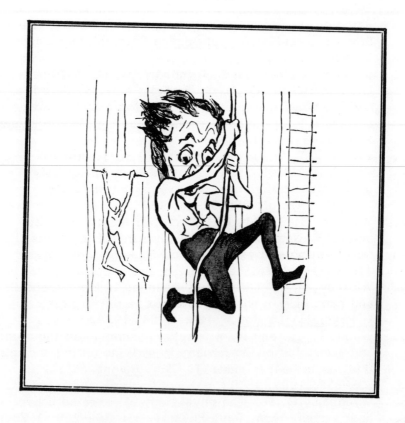

Thermal and Energetic Exchanges During Swimming

Ethan R. Nadel

During exercise, heat may be produced in the contracting muscles at rates up to fifteen or twenty times of the entire basal metabolic rate. Nearly all of this heat is rapidly removed from the muscles by the blood and transferred to the body core by the venous return to the heart. The brain then receives a representative sample of this warmed blood. Thermal receptors in specialized sites within the hypothalamus respond to the increased temperature and thereby (along with other relevant inputs, primarily those from the thermal receptors of the skin) trigger an integrated heat dissipation response, whereby heat is transferred to the skin via the bloodstream and removed from the body by physical means.

The above constitutes an abbreviated and simplified description of the events which lead up to the regulation of body temperature during exercise in air. However, this description does not adequately account for the occurrences during exercise in water. This is primarily due to the fact that water as a heat transfer medium places a much more severe thermal load on the body than does air of the same temperature. Water has a specific heat per unit volume of around 4000 times that of air and a thermal conductivity of around 25 times that of air. It is therefore predictable that the heat transfer characteristics of water should be considerably greater than those of air. Thus even when the body's heat production during vigorous swimming is up to fifteen times that during rest, if the heat loss to the environment is greater as it could well be during swimming in cold water, the internal body temperature would be gradually reduced to the point of interference with normal muscular activity. In the case of vigorous swimming in warm water, the water jacket around the individual prevents the evaporation of sweat, the primary means for dissipation of the body's excess heat. In this case, most of the heat production is stored within the body, resulting in a rapid increase in internal body temperature and, again, interferences with normal muscular activity. In the following paragraphs, the means by which heat is transferred from the body to the water are discussed. This discussion includes an analysis of the body's ability to modify the rate of heat flow by activating physiological responses.

The importance of an evaluation of heat transfer and thermoregulation during exercise in the water is evident to physiologists, but it is important from a practical viewpoint as well. In many parts of the world, divers are employed in tasks which may require extended bouts of swimming in water of extreme temperatures. In the case of accidental immersion, by shipwreck for instance, individuals may find themselves facing prolonged exposure in cold water. Channel swimmers are constantly searching for more efficient means of insulation against the cold water and competitive swimmers desirous of increasing performance consider that water temperature may be an important factor in gaining an extra second or two. Unfortunately, to this time there have been very few satisfactory attempts at analysis in these areas. This owes to difficulties in making measurements on humans while they are immersed or swimming. However, there have been several recent studies which have overcome many of these difficulties, and these will be elaborated upon in the following paragraphs.

The major thermal problems faced during swimming are these: is the thermoregulatory system capable of combatting the thermal physical aspects of a water environment in attempting to provide for an optimal internal body temperature? If the thermoregulatory system is capable of preventing excessive heat gain or loss in some conditions, at which combinations of swimming intensities and water temperatures does the thermoregulatory system become overwhelmed? And, finally, to what extent does the layer of subcutaneous body fat insulate the body against excessive heat transfer to the water?

It is well understood that the thermoregulatory system is sensitive to the thermal information both at the skin surface and within the body core. Lowered body temperatures result in peripheral vasoconstriction, which reduces the flow of blood (and therefore heat) from core to skin, from where the heat is transferred to the environment. The overall conductance (h_{sk}) of heat from core to skin is therefore an approximation of the skin blood flow and can be estimated as follows:

$$h_{sk} = (\underline{M} - \underline{E}_{res} - \underline{S}) \cdot (T_{in} - \bar{T}_{sk})^{-1} \qquad in \ W \cdot m^{-2} \cdot {}^{\circ}C^{-1}$$

$$(Eq \ 1)$$

where $\underline{M}$ = rate of metabolic heat production   in $W \cdot m^{-2}$

$\underline{E}_{res}$ = rate of respiratory evaporative heat loss
    in $W \cdot m^{-2}$

$\underline{S}$ = rate of storage of body heat   in $W \cdot m^{-2}$

T_{in} = internal body temperature   in °C

$\bar{T}_{sk}$ = average skin temperature   in °C

As has been discussed by many authors, the value of $\underline{S}$ is difficult to estimate, since one must have an approximation of the change of the average temperature of the body with time. There has been no universally acceptable technique for obtaining the average body temperature ($\bar{T}_b$), although it has been most frequently estimated as

$$\bar{T}_b = 0.7 \ T_{in} + 0.3 \ \bar{T}_{sk}$$

However, even if this were the optimal equation, other difficulties remain, such as obtaining the best approximation of T_{in}, especially during the rapid redistribution of body temperatures during the initial stages of water immersion. Thus, the best technique for estimating h_{sk} is when the body has obtained a thermal steady state and the value of $\underline{S} = 0$.

By transposing equation 1, we can arrive at the description of the transfer characteristic:

$$\underline{HF} = h_{sk} \ (T_{in} - \bar{T}_{sk}) \quad in \ W \cdot m^{-2} \qquad (Eq \ 2)$$

where $\underline{HF} = \underline{M} - \underline{E}_{res} - \underline{S}$ = heat flux to the skin

Therefore, the heat flux is a function of the core-to-skin thermal conductance and the temperature gradient between core and skin.

Although the overall conductance of heat from core to skin is variable, depending to a major extent on the information provided to the smooth muscle around the skin circulatory vessels from the thermoregulatory center, a portion of the overall conductance is invariant. This latter portion is a function of the density (or insulative component) of the tissues through which the heat flows. Thus, heat flux from the body core to the skin is comprised of a convective component, the heat carried by the blood through a variable resistance (the skin vessels, whose tone is under autonomic control), and a conductive component, the heat transferred across a fixed resistance. The latter is fixed in any individual and is largely determined by the thickness of the layer of subcutaneous body fat. Although muscular exercise has no direct effect upon the skin circulation, it may well increase local heat transfer from core to skin by increasing the local gradient of temperature in the region of the active tissues, as discussed in following paragraphs.

The heat transfer characteristics from skin to environment depend upon several factors. In an air environment heat can be transferred via radiation, convection and evaporation, as well as in the form of useful work. Thus the heat flux to the environment can be represented in the following manner.

$$\dot{HF} = W + [h_{r+c} (\bar{T}_{sk} - T_a) + h_e (P_{sk} - \phi P_a)] A_{D(eff)} \cdot A_D^{-1}$$
$$\text{in } W \cdot m^{-2} \cdot °C^{-1} \quad (Eq \ 3)$$

where W = rate of heat exchange by work, $W \cdot m^{-2}$

h_{r+c} = combined convective and radiative heat transfer coefficient, in $W \cdot m^{-2} \cdot °C^{-1}$

$\bar{T}_{sk}$ and T_a = mean skin and ambient temperatures, in °C

h_e = evaporative heat transfer coefficient, in $W \cdot m^{-2} \cdot mm \ Hg^{-1}$

ϕ = relative humidity, ND

P_{sk} and P_a = saturated water vapor pressures (mm Hg) at $\bar{T}_{sk}$ and T_a

$A_{D(eff)} \cdot A_D^{-1}$ = the fraction of the body surface area available for thermal exchanges, ND

In water, however, the equation becomes much simpler, because heat exchanges by radiation and evaporation are essentially nil, leaving convection as the only major avenue for the flux of heat. Since the useful work that can be accomplished in the water is also negligible and the effective surface area for exchange in nude humans in the water is nearly 1.00, the simplified description of the heat exchange in water becomes:

$$\underline{HF} = h_c \ (\bar{T}_{sk} - T_a) \hspace{3cm} (Eq \ 4)$$

It should be emphasized that for any ambient medium the convective heat transfer coefficient, h_c, describes the heat transfer characteristics of that medium and therefore serves to approximate the resistance to heat flow in given conditions. The value of h_c is fixed for given ambient conditions, being largely dependent upon such factors as the thermal conductivity and kinematic viscosity of the medium. However, the value of h_c in any medium is dependent to a certain extent upon the velocity of that medium. Thus, although the value of h_c may vary somewhat with the velocity in any environment, it is greatly different between water and air because of the differences in thermal physical properties between water and air. Accordingly, water has a much greater value of h_c than does air and offers practically no resistance to thermal exchange when compared to air. However, the heat flux from skin to water is dependent on the value of h_c multiplied by the thermal gradient between skin and water. Because of its high transfer coefficient, water offers practically no insulation at the skin-water interface and removes heat (if $T_{sk} > T_w$) rapidly. Hence, T_{sk} will be close to T_w and the product $h_c \cdot (\bar{T}_{sk} - T_w)$, or the heat flux from skin to water, need not be great. Nevertheless, the primary defense against heat flow from the body is described by equation 2 rather than equation 4, due to the extremely low resistance offered by the water.

Bullard and Rapp (3) recently described the heat exchanges in the water by use of a conceptual model similar to the one shown in Figure 1. In Figure 1, a simple schematic representation of the body demonstrates the various resistances to the flow of heat from the body core to the environment. Heat is produced in the body core as a by-product of the metabolic activities (eventually, all of the metabolism must be accounted for in the form of heat). The total metabolism includes the resting metabolism plus any additional metabolism which

$$h_{sk}\,(T_{in}-\bar{T}_{sk}) \quad = \quad h_e\,(P_{sk}-\phi P_a) + h_{r+c}\,(\bar{T}_{sk}-T_a)$$

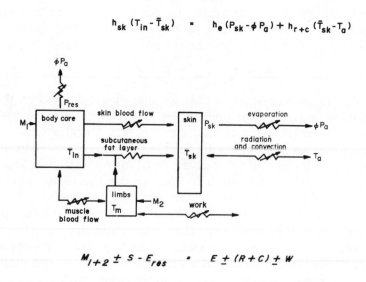

$$M_{1+2} \pm S - E_{res} \quad = \quad E \pm (R+C) \pm W$$

FIG. 1. *A simple conceptual model describing energy transfer from the body to the environment. The equation above the model describes the energy balance in heat transfer and temperature terms. The equation below the model describes the energy balance in the traditional manner.*

results from activities such as muscular contraction due to shivering or exercise. The body also contains heat stores which can be determined with a knowledge of the average tissue temperature of the body, the average specific heat of the tissues and the body mass. Heat flows down the thermal gradient at rates described by the various resistances to flow. Thus heat flows from the body core to the skin at a rate described by the product of the conductance and the core to skin thermal gradient, as indicated on the left of the top equation (from eq. 2) in Figure 1.

The conductance term (h_{sk}) of this equation is represented in the Figure by the two parallel resistances between core and skin. The resistance to heat flux offered by skin blood flow is adjustable; during conditions of low skin vascular resistance, there is a high flow of blood to the skin and therefore high conductance of heat from core-to-skin per unit of temperature difference. Conversely, increasing the skin vascular resistance causes the skin blood flow to be reduced, thereby reducing the heat conductance per degree of thermal gradient. The skin blood flow rate is under autonomic control and therefore depicted as an adjustable resistance. Conductance of heat is closely tied to the flow of blood because of the high specific heat of the blood (greater than 0.9 for most species). The fixed resistance to heat flow is a function of the thickness of the layer of subcutaneous body fat, which insulates the core from the skin. Fat is a relatively underperfused tissue, having a thermal conductivity of slightly less than 50 per cent that of muscle and around 35 per cent that of blood. The low thermal conductivity of fat and its insulating effect in water is not particularly a new observation, as Ishmael noted the following about 125 years ago:

> "For the whale is indeed wrapt up in
> his blubber as in a real blanket ....
> It is by reason of this cosy blanketing
> of his body that the whale is enabled
> to keep himself comfortable in all weathers,
> in all seas, times and tides .... How
> wonderful is it then —— except after explana-
> tion —— that this great monster, to whom
> corporeal warmth is as indispensable as it
> is to man; how wonderful that he should
> be found at home, immersed to his lips
> for life in those Arctic waters! "

Moby Dick, by Herman Melville

1850.

However, the understanding of the relative value of the insulative layer of fat during water immersion has been better understood and partially quantified in recent years.

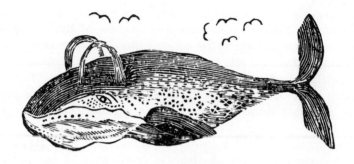

When the skin is maximally vasoconstricted, the value of the minimum conductance of heat is dependent to a great extent upon the thickness of the fat layer. The thicker the layer of insulative fat, the lower the rate of minimal heat conductance. This will be discussed in greater detail in following paragraphs.

The flow of heat from skin to environment is determined by the product of the relevant heat transfer coefficients and the skin to ambient gradient of water vapor pressure for evaporation and temperature for the so-called dry exchanges (radiation and convection). The sum of the rates of heat exchanged by evaporation and by radiation and convection in a given period must be equal to the amount of heat transferred from the core to the skin over the same period. This is shown in the top equation in Figure 1. The heat transfer coefficients are depicted as variable resistances because, although specific for a given ambient medium, they are related to the velocity of that medium, as discussed above. When the individual is in a water environment, the skin to water vapor pressure gradient is practically zero; hence, the product of the transfer coefficient and water vapor pressure gradient must be zero, and no heat can be dissipated by evaporation. This is also true in an air environment where the ambient vapor pressure is equal to or greater than that of the skin. Radiative exchanges in the water are minimal; thus, for practical purposes, we may consider that all heat transferred from skin to water is via convection (actually a small and constant component, 11 $W.m^{-2}.°C^{-1}$, is transferred by conduction (24)). However, this is usually incorporated into the convective term. In air the resistance to heat flow is relatively much greater than in water, because of differences in thermal physical properties as outlined above. Because of the high thermal transfer properties of water, the skin is brought close to the water temperature. As noted previously, the heat flux to the water (transfer coefficient times thermal gradient) is not as radically different between water and air as the difference between the thermal properties of these media would suggest.

The energy balance equation is shown on the bottom part of Fig. 1. During the thermal steady state at rest, the heat produced in the body by metabolism ($\underline{M}$), less the heat lost by evaporation ($\underline{E}_{res}$), is transferred through the skin to the environment via radiation ($\underline{R}$), convection ($\underline{C}$), and evaporation ($\underline{E}$) from the skin surface. In non-steady state conditions, where internal body temperature is changing, there is a change in the heat store of the body, and a storage term ($\underline{S}$) is added to the left side of the equation. During exercise some additional heat may be liberated to the environment or stored in the muscles in the form of useful work ($\underline{W}$). In the computation, all of the heat must be accounted for; hence, the two sides of the equation must balance.

In the following paragraphs, the topics which have been outlined above are discussed in detail. Since the primary concern of this discussion is thermal problems during swimming, a decided emphasis is placed upon studies of swimming. However, since detailed studies of swimmers are scarce, and since much of the information gathered from studies of immersion of humans at rest can be extrapolated to swimmers resting data will be referred to when appropriate.

Body Temperatures in the Water

A great deal of information is available concerning the changes in the body temperatures during rest and exercise in the water. The classic description of the channel swimmers by Pugh and Edholm (23) provide the reader with an entertaining and informative insight into the value of insulation during extended exposures. Their primary studies were on two

swimmers, J. Z. 164 cm in height, 96 kg in weight, and G.P.,
183 cm in height, 75 kg in weight. Subject J. Z. could regu-
larly tolerate swimming in 15°C water for up to 7 hours without a decrease in rectal temperature. He was characterized
as "...in good condition and he ran up the beach" following
the extended swim. It was also noted that his "... forearms
and legs were intensely pale; his brachial pulse was only
felt with difficulty, and his radial pulse was impalpable until
50 minutes later." These observations indicated that this subject was able to restrict blood flow (and, hence, heat flow) to
the periphery to a very great extent. Furthermore, the combination of the minimal blood flow and the high amount of subcutaneous fat provided this subject with an impressive insulative
capability. In comparison, subject G. P. could not stand after
leaving the water following only 30 minutes of swimming. At
this time his rectal temperature had fallen to 34.5°C from
37.0°C and he was shivering violently. It is clear from these
observations that the decrease in internal body temperature
during swimming in cold water was inversely related to the
amount of body fat.

Sloan and Keatinge (28) studied the changes in oral temperature in young (8-19 years of age) male and female subjects
swimming between 18 and 40 min in a pool of 20°C. Swimming
speed was 30 m.min^{-1}. Major decreases in oral temperature
were observed, particularly in 5 males between 8 and 15 years,
who had low body weights and low subscapular fat thicknesses.
These subjects all had oral temperatures below 35° at the end
of swim, with a maximal decrease in temperature of 3.2°C.
There was a linear relationship between the rate of decrease
of oral temperature and the mean normalized (for surface to
volume differences) reciprocal fat thickness of their subjects.
This finding is not too surprising, since when exercising in a
given water temperature at a given metabolic rate, the energy
exchange should be dependent to a large extent on the amount
of insulation of the subject (the fixed resistance, as discussed
previously).

Perhaps the most complete study of the changes in internal
body temperature during swimming was in the recent report of
Holmér and Bergh (10). They studied five subjects who swam
at submaximal (50% $\dot{V}O_2$ max) and maximal levels in water temperatures of 18°, 26° and 34°C. These subjects varied in body
fat content between 4 and 12 percent and skinfold thickness
from 5.3 to 14.0 min. Measurements of esophageal tempera-

ture were made continuously during swimming and therefore
this report was able to provide not only the change of internal
temperature with time, but the pattern of change as well.
Holmér and Bergh found that 4 out of the 5 subjects underwent
a decrease in T_{es} during 20 min of submaximal swim in 18°C
water, with the amount of decrease inversely proportional to
the skinfold thickness (Fig. 2). The maximum decrease (in the
subject with the lowest skinfold thickness) was 1.6°C.

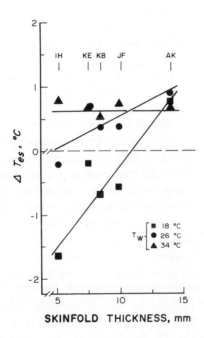

FIG. 2. *The change in internal (esophageal) tem-*
perature as related to skinfold thickness in five
subjects after 20 min of submaximal swimming in
18, 26 and 34°C water. Modified from Holmér and
Bergh (10).

Further, the rate of decrease of T_{es} in this subject was constant at 0.08°C per min over the entire 20 min period. In the 26°C water, swimming at 50% $\dot{V}O_2$ max allowed the subjects to maintain nearly a constant T_{es} over the 20 min period, with an average increase of only 0.3°C. Again the only subject of the 5 to suffer a decrease in T_{es} in 26°C water was the one with the lowest skinfold thickness. As in the 18°C water, the change in T_{es} was related to skinfold thickness. In fact, there was a linear relationship between change in T_{es} and skinfold thickness at any water temperature after 20 min of submaximal swim, with the slope of this relationship steeper in the colder water. In the 34°C water, the average increase in T_{es} was around 0.7°C. Previously, Nadel, et al (19) had shown that all 3 of their subjects underwent decreases in T_{es} after 20 min of swimming in 18°C and 26°C water at 40% $\dot{V}O_2$ max, but in the 26°C water at 70% $\dot{V}O_2$ max, the subjects showed slight (2) or major (1) increases in T_{es}. Their subjects increased T_{es} in 33°C water by around 1.0°C after 20 min of swimming at 40% $\dot{V}O_2$ max and by around 1.5°C after 20 min at 70% $\dot{V}O_2$ max. Thus, it may be concluded that the rate and amount of internal temperature change is a complex function of the water temperature, swimming speed and skinfold thickness.

The data correlating the fall in internal temperature with the reciprocal of mean skinfold thickness during swimming at a given metabolic rate and in a given water temperature directly follow an accumulation of similar results obtained for resting subjects (25). Perhaps the most important variable in these studies is the maintenance of the metabolic rate, because as internal temperature falls, the metabolic rate tends to increase during rest (21) as well as during swimming (10). Therefore, a portion of the error in the correlation between fall in internal temperature and reciprocal of mean skinfold thickness is the result of the body's attempt to prevent the fall of internal temperature by increasing its metabolism ... however, the cooling effects of the water exceed the body's ability to thermoregulate in these extreme conditions.

The change in the temperatures of the skin differ slightly between rest in still water and swimming, but in either case skin temperatures are always higher than water temperature when the latter does not exceed 35°C. This is perfectly predictable, since heat flows down the temperature gradient from skin to water in the transfer from the body to the environment. Many investigators have approximated skin temperature as equal to water temperature in their studies. However, these approximations can be up to 2°C in error under some conditions.

Nadel, et al (19) measured skin temperatures at four skin surface sites during rest and swimming exposures to 18°, 26° and 33°C water. The technique employed was affixing a thermocouple to the skin under a strip of surgical tape. The heat transfer coefficient of the tape was calculated to be two orders of magnitude greater than that of the skin, thereby offering practically no insulation at the skin-to-water interface. They found that mean skin temperatures ($\bar{T}_{sk}$) were related to both water temperature (T_w) and water velocity during rest and to T_w during swimming. During rest in still water $\bar{T}_{sk}$ was about 2.0°C higher than T_w in the 18°C water, about 1.0°C higher than T_w in 26°C water and only about 0.2°C higher in 33°C water. When the water was moving by the resting subject, the skin-to-water temperature gradient was always less than 1.0°C and was greater in the colder water. During swimming the $\bar{T}_{sk} - T_w$ gradient ranged between 0.2 - 0.4°C in the 33°C water to 0.5 - 0.9°C in the 18°C water. Swimming speed did not appear to have an important influence on $\bar{T}_{sk}$.

It is important to note that, even though skin temperatures are close to the water temperature, there is a difference between the two. Therefore, when using water temperature as an approximation of $\bar{T}_{sk}$, it is important to realize that they are not precisely the same. This is particularly important when using water as a means to clamp $\bar{T}_{sk}$ in studies of thermoregulation. Moving water, such as occurs when the subject is shivering, can markedly alter the $\bar{T}_{sk} - T_w$ gradient, bringing $\bar{T}_{sk}$ closer to T_w. Conversely, when a subject is resting quietly in still water, the $\bar{T}_{sk} - T_w$ gradient may be between 1.0 and 2.0°C, depending upon T_w.

Energy Losses to the Water

The evaluation of the energy losses from skin to water depends upon the determination of the convective heat transfer coefficient (h_c) of the skin in both still and moving water and during swimming at different speeds. The heat transfer coefficient provides the rate of heat flux from skin to water per degree of thermal gradient.

Direct measurement of h_c in humans during swimming has been difficult to make. Rapp (24) and Witherspoon, et al (31) made theoretical analyses based upon heat transfer theory in the former case and measurements with a copper manikin as well in the latter. Rapp's calculations were based upon information from air exposures and differences between water and air in thermal physical properties. His analysis provides a value of $h_c = 94$ W.m^{-2}.°C^{-1} during rest in still water and $h_c = 400$ W.m^{-2}.°C^{-1} during swimming at 0.5 m.s^{-1}. By adjusting (19) for his underestimates in metabolic rate at the conditions he uses (22°C water), we arrive at revised values of h_c of 172 W.m^{-2}.°C^{-1} for rest and 459 W.m^{-2}.°C^{-1} during swimming. Witherspoon, et al measured values of h_c of 137 W.m^{-2}.°C^{-1} in still water and 588 W.m^{-2}.°C^{-1} in water moving at 0.5 m.s^{-1}, values reasonably close to those predicted by Rapp.

The only direct measurements of h_c that have been made during swimming were reported by Nadel, et al (19). They used copper-tellurium heat flow discs to estimate the heat flux across the skin and a swimming flume (1) to enable them to make continuous measurements of heat flow, $\bar{T}_{sk}$ and T_w during swimming. By relating mean weighted heat flow to the $T_{sk} - T_w$ gradient at different water temperatures, they found values of h_c of 230 W.m^{-2}.°C^{-1} for subjects resting in still water and 580 W.m^{-2}.°C^{-1} for subjects swimming at speeds between 0.50 and 0.95 m.s^{-1} (Fig. 3). The latter finding, that h_c was independent of water velocity, was surprising, because in air h_c is dependent to a certain extent upon the air velocity (15, 22). However, during swimming, the independence of h_c from water velocity was likely the consequence of the high degree of water turbulence around the subject. That is to say that the effective water velocity around the body was probably similar between swimming speeds of 0.50 and 0.95 m.s^{-1}. The measured values of h_c in these studies were relatively similar to those predicted by Rapp (24) and measured from a manikin by Witherspoon, et al (31), although Witherspoon, et al showed a much higher h_c value for a higher water velocity. However, the manikin was not creating the turbulence around its body by swimming motions and this may account for part of the difference.

It is noteworthy that indirect calorimetric calculations, using $\underline{M} - \underline{E}_{res} - \underline{S}$ as the measure of heat flux in the same study (19), provided nearly an identical value of h_c during swimming. This value was 630 W.m^{-2}.°C^{-1} compared with 580 W.m^{-2}.°C^{-1} obtained from the heat flow discs. However, during rest in still water indirect calorimetry gave a marked

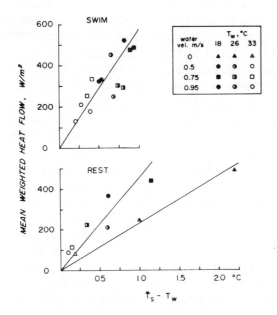

FIG. 3. Mean weighted heat flow in three subjects as a function of skin-to-water temperature gradient. The slope of each relation is the convective heat transfer coefficient. From Nadel, et al (19), with permission of the American Physiological Society.

underestimate of the h_c value obtained with heat flow discs. This is probably the result of the difficulty in the determination of $\underline{S}$ in resting subjects. Recently, Smith and Hanna (29) exposed 14 subjects to a 3 hour water immersion with a water velocity of around 0.05 m. s^{-1} (not quite still). Using their steady state data (when $\underline{S} = 0$) and the $\bar{T}_{sk} - T_w$ gradient that has been observed in 33°C water (19), we estimate a value of

h_c of between 300–400 $W.m^{-2}.°C^{-1}$ for resting subjects in
slightly moving water. This is slightly greater than Nadel,
et al (19) found for subjects in still water, but slightly
less than they found in moving water. It is probably very
difficult to estimate $\underline{S}$ during conditions of significant redistribution of body heat from the subcutaneous zone into the
body core during the transient of cold water immersion (5).
During an extended steady state or during swimming, however,
the body is well-stirred and the discrepancy between the value
of h_c calculated from indirect calorimetric analysis and that
calculated from the heat flow measurements was minimal.

In conclusion, the skin to water interface offers very
little resistance to heat flow. This means that practically all
of the heat brought to the skin surface is rapidly transferred to
the water. The rate of transfer is described by the heat transfer coefficient and the $\bar{T}_{sk} - T_w$ gradient. Since the value of
h_c is about 200 times that in air, it can be seen that heat transfer in water is considerably greater than in air, even considering the smaller thermal gradients between skin and water. Thus,
in order to conserve body heat in the water, the object is to
keep the body heat away from the skin. It should be emphasized that the heat transfer coefficient during swimming is 2.5
to 3 times that during rest in still water but only 1.5 times
that during rest in moving water. Since the relative values of
h_c are high in either case, heat transfer from skin to water is
not appreciably increased during swimming as compared to
floating in moving water.

Energy Production During Swimming

Technically, it has been a difficult problem to measure the
oxygen uptake of a swimming human. This is easy to understand; a swimmer does not easily avail himself to the carrying
of probes or mouthpieces or Douglas bags or any other necessary equipment to collect samples of expired air. Thus, a few
unique solutions have provided the sparse data that has become
available.

Several investigators (4, 13) tethered their subjects in
water in an attempt to simulate swimming and made measurements from individuals pulling against the tether. Increased
exercise intensities were produced by increasing stroke frequency. This technique provided the experimenter with the
ability to obtain measurements, since the subject was

stationary during exercise, but, unfortunately, provided only an approximation of the true events during swimming, since increased stroke frequency was not accompanied by increased water resistance.

Karpovich and Millman (12) examined the metabolic cost of swimming by requiring their subjects to swim while holding their breath. They then measured the oxygen debt during an extended recovery period. This technique provided them with extraordinarily high values of $\dot{V}O_2$, or the order of 20 to 30 liters . min^{-1} for maximal swimming. Needless to say, this is not the technique of choice.

McCardle, et al (14) studied ventilatory exchanges during swimming by suspending gas collection equipment from an aluminum pole and following the subject by walking on the side of the pool as the subject swam. This was a reasonable solution, although it is not known whether the subject was restricted by the apparatus. Exercise intensity in this study was modified by altering stroke frequency although it is common knowledge that competitive swimmers generally tend to increase speed by increasing the pulling power rather than stroke frequency. However, the metabolic result is probably relatively similar, barring drastic changes in efficiency. Oxygen uptake was found to be essentially linear with stroke frequency (swimming speed) during the 4-min swims.

DiPrampero, et al (7) attempted to simulate natural movements by having their subjects swim in a circular pool, with gas collection apparati suspended from a platform which was moveable alongside the edge of the pool and which served as a pacing device for the subject. Their primary goal was an analysis of the relation between energy expenditure and drag during swimming. They found that the energy expenditure at a given swimming speed was a linear function of the total drag the swimmer had to overcome. They further reported that the energy cost of swimming a given distance $(\dot{V}O_2 \cdot v^{-1})$ was independent of swimming velocity for the two velocities studied (0.55 and 0.90 $m.s^{-1}$), due to the constancy in the efficiency to drag ratio over this range of velocities. Unfortunately, they did not examine the effect of water temperature on this relation. This would have been interesting to determine whether the increased metabolism of swimming in cold water could partially be attributed to a reduction of the efficiency to drag ratio because of increased water viscosity (this will be discussed in greater detail below).

In 1972 Astrand and Englesson (1) described the development and installation of a swimming flume. This swimming
flume made it possible to study the physiological and biome-
chanical aspects of swimming under conditions practically identical with open water. The subject is able to swim in the flowing water and keeps his or her position constant in the basin.
In this respect the swimming flume is analogous to the motor
driven treadmill. In the basin water is circulated in a 2.5 m
wide, 1.2 m deep vertical loop. Water speed can be accurately
controlled between 0 and 2.00 $m.s^{-1}$ ($\pm$ 0.02 $m.s^{-1}$). Water
temperature can also be varied between 10 and 40°C, and control achieved ($\pm$ 0.5°C) due to the inertia of the water mass
(38×10^3 ℓ) and by visual monitoring of water temperature and
making manual adjustments. Thus, the swimmer can be subjected to a wide variety of conditions and yet be accessible
for attachment of probes or sampling of blood or expired air.
The development of the swimming flume was surely a milestone
for the study of the physiological events during swimming.

Holmer (9) used the swimming flume in his analysis of the
oxygen uptake of swimmers of different sex and class while
performing different strokes. Water temperature was 26°C. He
found that $\dot{V}O_2$ differed at a given swimming speed according
to the stroke employed ($\dot{V}O_2$ was related to the efficiency of
the stroke). $\dot{V}O_2$ tended to be linear with swimming velocity
at low velocities, but tended to increase per unit of velocity
at near maximal levels. This has been explained as the result
of a decrease in the efficiency of swimming in the presence of
increasing drag (7).

Also using the swimming flume, Nadel, et al (19) examined
the cost of swimming at different velocities and at different
water temperatures. $\dot{V}O_2$ was found to be approximately linearly related to swimming velocity at submaximal levels at a
given water temperature. However, $\dot{V}O_2$ was greater in 18°C
water than in 26°C water during rest and during swimming at
any submaximal swimming intensity, with the increment in $\dot{V}O_2$
in 18°C water being 400 - 500 $ml.min^{-1}$. Furthermore, $\dot{V}O_2$ in
26°C water tended to be 200 - 300 $ml.min^{-1}$ higher than
when swimming at submaximal levels in 33°C water. (Fig. 4).
The increment in $\dot{V}O_2$ between 26° and 18°C water was necessary to support the considerable shivering contractions superimposed upon the contractions due to swimming alone. The
shivering response was the result of the lowered T_{sk} and T_{es}.
This increment was the same during rest and during swimming,

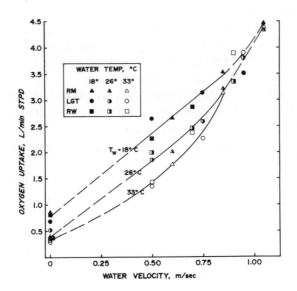

FIG. 4.   Oxygen uptake as a function of water velocity (swimming speed) when swimming in 18, 26
and 33°C water.   From Nadel, et al (19), with permission of the American Physiological Society.

indicating that the shivering was maintained at a relatively
constant rate during swimming. This phenomenon has been
observed during bicycle ergometer exercise with lowered internal body temperatures as well (20). The constancy of the increment during rest and exercise, the visible and violent shivering contractions during swimming and the fact of similar observations of the increased metabolism of shivering during exercise in air constitute indirect evidence against the concept
of the increased metabolism in the cold water being the result
of the increased viscosity of the water. However, the efficiency to drag ratio may have also been reduced due to the move-

ments of shivering. It is clear that the increased metabolism of these subjects swimming in cold water represents an attempt at thermoregulation. As noted in a preceding section, all of these subjects had very low body temperatures. The increased metabolism during swimming in cold water was not sufficient to raise internal body temperature in subjects whose rates of heat transfer from body core to the water exceeded the rates of heat production even when the latter was elevated. However, increased metabolism does prevent internal body temperature from decreasing at a greater rate.

Holmér and Bergh (10) made similar observations in 4 out of 5 subjects (the 5th subject was the fattest, with an average skinfold thickness of 14 mm). During submaximal swimming at a given speed, these subjects showed a linear relation between increased $\dot{V}O_2$ and lowered T_{es} below a T_{es} threshold of about 37.2°C (Fig. 5). Thus, the body attempts to counter-

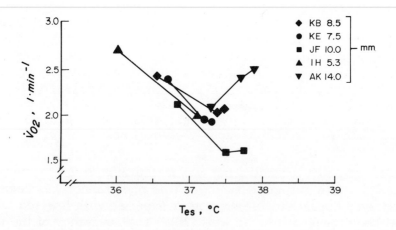

FIG. 5. *Oxygen uptake relation to internal tem-*
perature during submaximal swimming. Subjects'
skinfold thicknesses in mm appear in upper right.
Modified from Holmér and Bergh (10).

act the stress of cold by increasing $\dot{V}O_2$, and therefore heat production, as it senses the lowered body temperatures. The linear relation between the change of metabolism with respect to the change in T_{es} is described as continuous proportional control. This relation is qualitatively similar to the mechanism described for the control of shivering in humans (2, 10, 20, 21), the control of sweating during rest and exercise (18) and the control of skin blood flow during rest and exercise (30).

Generally speaking, swimmers are not able to achieve their maximum levels of $\dot{V}O_2$ in water of 18°C, and even at water of 26°C lean subjects, who undergo decreases in internal body temperature while swimming, fall short of the maximal value that they are able to achieve in 33°C water. The two lean subjects in the Nadel, et al (19) study were only able to reach 85% of maximal aerobic power in 18°C water and 92% in 26°C water, compared to their performance in 33°C water. In 18°C water both of these subjects had T_{es} values below 36.0°C at the termination of the swim. They complained of an inability to contract their muscles and of muscle fatigue rather than cardio-respiratory distress as the primary cause of fatigue. This observation was confirmed by Holmér and Bergh (10), who found comparatively low muscle temperatures following maximal swims in 18°C water. They concluded that low muscle temperatures affect such chemical and physical processes as enzyme activity and diffusion rate at the cellular level. Thus, reduced maximal performance in cold water is likely the direct result of the effect of cold upon local muscular activities. However, maximal heart rate values (but not necessarily cardiac output values) were also lower in colder water during maximal swims (10, 19), suggesting that there may be important central effects of cold as well.

Conductance of Heat From Body Core to Skin

Because of the very high coefficient of heat transfer between skin and water, the major defense against excessive heat loss while swimming is by minimizing the conduction of heat from core to skin. By reducing skin blood flow to minimal values, the rate of heat transfer from core to skin is reduced to a rate dependent upon the value of the fixed resistance (see Fig. 1), thereby reducing the $\bar{T}_{sk}$ and, therefore, the $\bar{T}_{sk}$ to T_w gradient and the total heat flux.

There have been a number of studies which have reported

an inverse relation between the critical water temperature for increased heat production, which has been said to represent the level of maximal insulation (minimal conductance) for an individual (25), to the individual's subcutaneous fat layer. The critical water temperature (T_{cw}) has been generally defined as the lowest water temperature a subject can tolerate for 3 h without shivering (11, 26). Recently, however, the T_{cw} has been slightly re-defined by a linear approximation method, which accounts for non-shivering increases in metabolic rate (29). The latter has the advantage in that it is somewhat more analytical and less subjective. In using the "old" T_{cw} to derive maximum body insulation, Hong (11) recently reported the cumulative data from a number of previous studies (89 subjects), which showed a positive correlation between maximum body insulation and subcutaneous fat thickness. This confirms what was deduced from the data of Pugh and Edholm (23); the thicker the underperfused layer of fat, the greater the insulative value. Using the "new" T_{cw}, Smith and Hanna (29) confirmed this finding and added the notion of using water/air core-to-environment conductance ratios as an index of the insulative capacity of the subject. Accordingly, the thicker the skinfold, the lower the water to air conductance ratio. These ratios ranged from 2.3 to 4.4 in their study, indicating that the combined heat transfer characteristic from core-to-environment was as little as 2.3 times greater in water than in air of any given temperature and velocity in a relatively fat subject and 4.4 times greater in a relatively lean subject. They further calculated the minimal conductance values at any given mean skinfold thickness for resting conditions. This relationship was described by a hyperbola, with values of minimal conductance of 12 and 6 $W.m^{-2}.°C^{-1}$ for mean skinfold thicknesses of 5 and 20 mm. These observations underline the fact that the extremely high heat transfer coefficient of the skin in a water environment does not imply that heat loss much be equally as high, because the heat loss is a function of the heat transfer coefficient and the skin to water thermal gradient. Thus, when the gradient is relatively low, the heat flux may also be relatively low. Molnar (17) pointed this out about 30 years ago and Gagge (8) discussed this type of problem nearly 40 years ago.

The reduction of the heat flux from core to skin to water is achieved physiologically by reducing peripheral blood flow to rates less than 0.5 $ml.min^{-1}.100$ ml tissue^{-1} in water temperatures at or below T_{cw}. This is true for resting conditions. Bullard and Rapp (3) have pointed out that, to attain tissue conductances on the order of 6 $W.m^{-2}.°C^{-1}$, either a subcutaneous fat layer of 3 cm in thickness or 6 cm of thickness of bloodless muscle would be required. Rennie's data (25) show that fat can only account for about 50% of the total insulation. The inference of Bullard and Rapp's discussion is that in addition to the reduction in blood flow to the periphery, the body core restricts heat loss by shifting venous return to deep veins, thereby establishing a counter-current heat exchanger whereby heat is transferred directly from arterial blood to the venous blood returning to the core. However, Mitchell, et al (16) have calculated that a counter-current mechanism is not necessary to conserve heat in humans during cold air exposure. Although it is well established physiologically and anatomically that porpoises use this technique for heat conservation during prolonged dives in cold water (27), the presence of counter-current heat exchange in humans is still an open question.

During swimming, the oxygen demands of the contracting muscle preclude minimal blood flow. Therefore, it should not be possible to maintain peripheral blood flow at rates as low as 0.5 $ml.min^{-1}$. 100 ml tissue during swimming. Nadel, et al (19) have reported h_{sk} values that ranged from 14-22 $W.m^{-2}.°C^{-1}$ during swimming at 0.50 $m.s^{-1}$ in 18°C water; these are on the order of 3 to 5 times the minimal values during rest. When their subjects swam at a velocity of 0.75 $m.s^{-1}$, h_{sk} values were even higher (ranging from 21-31 $W.m^{-2}.°C^{-1}$), reflecting the greater oxygen, and therefore circulatory demands of the contracting muscles. During swims in the 33°C, values of h_{sk} were considerably higher, ranging between 35 and 45 $W.m^{-2}.°C^{-1}$, when T_{es} was low (36.5°C), to between 85 and 95 $W.m^{-2}.°C^{-1}$ when T_{es} was high (37.9°C). The curvilinear relation between h_{sk} and T_{es} (Figure 6) indicates that, above the blood flow to the contracting muscles to satisfy metabolic demands, there was also a regulated blood flow to the skin in response to the thermoregulatory demands.

In the cold water it is likely that the increased (above minimal) h_{sk} values were the result of the increased conductive transfer of heat across the muscle - skin gradient, since T_m was elevated during swimming (10) as a result of increased muscle blood flow and/or increased local heat production. Thus, referring back to Fig. 1, the primary increase in h_{sk}

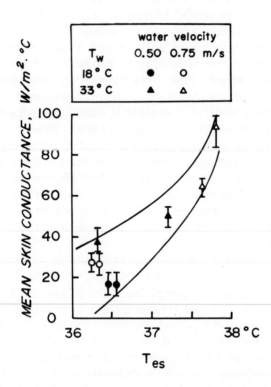

FIG. 6. Mean (± range) skin conductance of three
subjects as a function of internal temperature
when swimming in cold (18°C) and warm (33°C) water.
From Nadel, et al (19), with permission of the
American Physiological Society.

during swimming is a result of increased heat transfer across
the fixed resistance. As the body stores heat, as occurs when
swimming in 33°C water, increased levels of T_{es} and $\bar{T}_{sk}$
stimulate active vasodilation in the skin, thereby reducing the
core-to-skin thermal gradient and increasing the conductance
of heat from core-to-skin.

The effect of different insulative layers of body fat upon

heat exchange is readily seen in Table 1. Using representative data gathered from different sources (3, 10, 19, 24, 29), a hypothetical energy balance is constructed for two individuals, one with a skinfold thickness of 5 mm and the other with a skinfold of 20 mm. These subjects are placed at rest in still water and during swimming at water velocities of 0.50 and 0.75 m.s^{-1} at a water temperature of 18°. It is clear that the lean individual is at a considerable disadvantage insofar as his capabilities for maintaining internal body temperature are concerned. In each case, the lean individual suffers a considerable decrease in internal temperature while the individual with a moderate level of subcutaneous fat is able to resist a decrease. Curiously, the lower rate of swimming is optimal for the lean individual in attempting to prevent excessive heat loss. This is probably explained by the inability to produce enough heat by shivering to balance heat loss during rest and the relatively high skin conductances (both convective and conductive transfer) during fairly intense swimming. Apparently, the combination of lower skin conductances and a relatively higher metabolism during moderate swimming provides for a halving of the net rate of heat flux when compared to rest in still water or fairly intense swimming. However, even a halving of the net heat flux merely extends the swimming time from one hour to two hours before internal body temperature is decreased to levels which are prohibitive to continued performance.

The major conclusion that can be drawn about thermoregulation during swimming is that the thermal physical properties of the water environment are such as to override the body's capabilities for thermoregulation in extreme conditions. Because of the body's thermal inertia, the time of exposure is important. This is especially true for extended (more than 20-30 min) exposure. However, the thickness of the insulative layer of body fat is the single most important factor in determining the rate of heat flux. This was well demonstrated in the Pugh and Edholm study (23) and, recently, quantified to some extent by Smith and Hanna (29) and Holmér and Bergh (10). That the body attempts to regulate its internal temperature during swimming is clearly illustrated in Figures 5 and 6, where a proportional effector system response is made to a change in internal temperature. However, that the body is unable to regulate well in extreme water temperatures is apparent from the data of Table 1. The thermoregulatory

TABLE I

A theoretical energy balance for two individuals at rest and swimming in 18°C water. The two individuals have 5 mm and 20 mm skinfold thicknesses, respectively. Terms are defined in the text.

$T_w = 18°C$

	h_{sk} ***	$T_{in} - \bar{T}_{sk}$ *	HF **	h_c ***	$\bar{T}_{sk} - T_w$ *	$\bar{M}$ **	M_{req} **	$\underline{S}$ **	$\Delta T_{in} \cdot hr^{-1}$ *
Rest									
5 mm	12	19	228	230	1.00	138	240	-102	-1.82
20 mm	6	19	114	230	0.50	138	125	13	0.23
Swim 0.50 m.s⁻¹									
5 mm	22	19	418	580	0.72	397	450	-53	-0.95
20 mm	14	19	268	580	0.46	397	300	97	1.74
Swim 0.75 m.s⁻¹									
5 mm	31	19	589	580	1.02	519	630	-111	-1.98
20 mm	21	19	399	580	0.69	519	441	78	1.39

*** $W \cdot m^{-2} \cdot °C^{-1}$
** $W \cdot m^{-2}$
* °C

mechanism is an extremely effective one in air .... the thermal
physical properties of water are sufficient to override thermoregulation in individuals who lack the necessary layer of insulative fat. Thus, to return to the observations of Ishmael:

> ".... herein we see the rare virtue
> of .... thick walls and the rare
> virtue of interior spaciousness. Oh, man!
> Admire and model thyself after
> the whale! Do thou too remain
> warm among ice .... keep they blood
> fluid at the Pole .... retain,
> O man! in all seasons a temperature
> of thine own."

Moby Dick, by Herman Melville

1850.

References

1.   Astrand, P.-O., and S. Englesson. A swimming flume.
     J. Appl. Physiol. 33: 514, 1972.
2.   Benzinger, T. H., C. Kitzinger and A. W. Pratt. The
     human thermostat. In: Temperature, Its Measurement
     and Control in Science and Industry, J. D. Hardy (Ed.).
     New York, Reinhold, 1963, Vol. 3, part 3, pp. 637-665.
3.   Bullard, R. W., and G. M. Rapp. Problems of body
     heat loss in water immersion. Aerospace Med. 41: 1269-
     1277, 1970.
4.   Costill, D. L., P. J. Cahill, and D. Eddy. Metabolic
     responses to submaximal exercise in three water tem-
     peratures. J. Appl. Physiol. 22: 628-632, 1967.
5.   Craig, A. B., Jr., and M. Dvorak. Heat balance during
     head out immersion in water (Abstract). Federation Proc.
     32: 391, 1973.
6.   Davies, M., B. Ekblom, U. Bergh and I.-L. Kanstrup-
     Jensen. The effects of hypothermia on submaximal and
     maximal work performance. Acta Physiol. Scand. 95:
     201-202, 1975.

7. DiPrampero, P. E., D. R. Pendergast, D. W. Wilson and D. W. Rennie. Energetics of swimming in man. J. Appl. Physiol. 37: 1-5, 1974.

8. Gagge, A. P. Standard operative temperature, a generalized temperature scale, applicable to direct and partitional calorimetry. Am. J. Physiol. 131: 93-103, 1940.

9. Holmér, I. Oxygen uptake during swimming in man. J. Appl. Physiol. 33: 502-509, 1972.

10. Holmér, I. and U. Bergh. Metabolic and thermal response to swimming in water at various temperatures. J. Appl. Physiol. 37: 702-705, 1974.

11. Hong, S. K. Pattern of cold adaptation in women divers of Korea (ama). Fed. Proc. 32: 1614-1622, 1973.

12. Karpovich, P. V., and N. Millman. Energy expenditure in swimming. Am. J. Physiol. 142: 140-144, 1944.

13. Magel, J. R. and J. A. Faulkner. Maximum oxygen uptakes of college swimmers. J. Appl. Physiol. 22: 929-933, 1967.

14. McArdle, W. D., R. M. Glaser, and J. R. Magel. Metabolic and cardiorespiratory response during free swimming and treadmill walking. J. Appl. Physiol. 30: 733-738, 1971.

15. Mitchell, D., C. H. Wyndham, A. J. Vermeulen, T. Hodgson, A. R. Atkins and H. S. Hofmeyr. Radiant and convective heat transfer of nude men in dry air. J. Appl. Physiol. 26: 111-118, 1969.

16. Mitchell, J. W. and G. W. Myers. An analytical model of counter-current heat exchange phenomena. Biophys. J. 8: 897-911, 1968.

17. Molnar, G. W. Survival of hypothermia by men immersed in the ocean. J. Am. Med. Assoc. 131: 1046-1050, 1946.

18. Nadel, E. R., R. W. Bullard and J. A. J. Stolwijk. Importance of skin temperature in the regulation of sweating. J. Appl. Physiol. 31: 80-87, 1971.

19. Nadel, E. R., I. Holmér, U. Bergh, P.-O. Astrand, and J. A. J. Stolwijk. Energy exchanges of swimming man. J. Appl. Physiol. 36: 465-471, 1974.

20. Nadel, E. R., I. Holmér, U. Bergh, P.-O. Astrand and J. A. J. Stolwijk. Thermoregulatory shivering during exercise. Life Sci. 13: 983-989, 1973.

21.   Nadel, E. R. and S. M. Horvath. Optimal evaluation of cold tolerance in man. In: Comparative Studies of Human Adaptability of Japanese, Caucasians and Japanese Americans. S. M. Horvath, S. Kondo, H. Matsui and H. Yoshimura (Eds.) Univ. of Tokyo Press, Tokyo, 1975, pp. 89-117.

22.   Nishi, Y., and A. P. Gagge. Direct evaluation of convective heat transfer coefficient by naphthalene sublimation. J. Appl. Physiol. 29: 830-838, 1970.

23.   Pugh, L. G. C., and O. G. Edholm. The physiology of channel swimmers. Lancet 2: 761-768, 1955.

24.   Rapp, G. M. Convection coefficients of man in a forensic area of thermal physiology: heat transfer in underwater exercise. J. Physiol., Paris 63: 392-396, 1971.

25.   Rennie, D. W. Thermal insulation of Korean diving women and non-divers in water. In: Physiology of Breath-Hold Diving and the Ama of Japan, edited by H. Rahn and T. Yokoyama. Publ. 1341 NAS-NRC, Washinton, D. C., 1965, p. 315-324.

26.   Rennie, D. W., B. G. Covino, B. J. Howell, S. H. Song, B. S. Kang, and S. K. Hong. Physical insulation of Korean diving women. J. Appl. Physiol. 17: 961-966, 1962.

27.   Scholander, P. F., R. Hock, V. Walters, F. Johnson, and L. Irving. Heat regulation in some arctic and tropical mammals and birds. Biol. Bull. 99: 237-258, 1950.

28.   Sloan, R. E. G. and W. R. Keatinge. Cooling rates of young people swimming in cold water. J. Appl. Physiol. 35: 371-375, 1973.

29.   Smith, R. M. and J. M. Hanna. Skinfolds and resting heat loss in cold air and water: temperature equivalence. J. Appl. Physiol. 39: 93-102, 1975.

30.   Wenger, C. B., M. F. Roberts, J. A. J. Stolwijk and E. R. Nadel. Forearm blood flow during body temperature transients produced by leg exercise. J. Appl. Physiol. 38: 58-63, 1975.

31.   Witherspoon, J. M., R. F. Goldman, and J. R. Breckenridge. Heat transfer coefficients of humans in cold water. J. Physiol. Paris 63: 459-462, 1971.

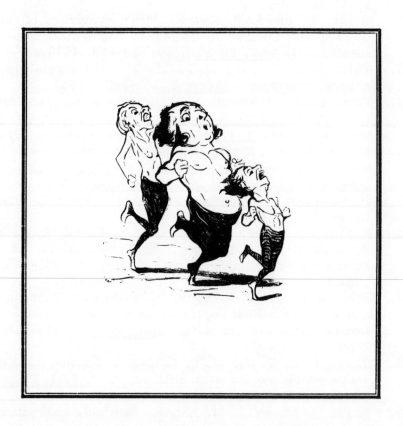

A Brief Summary...

Ethan R. Nadel and Steven M. Horvath

The discussions in the previous chapters constitute an up-to-date analysis of the workings of the temperature regulatory system in humans during exercise. However, despite their thoroughness, there are a number of questions that have not been satisfactorily dealt with, primarily because of the paucity of information that exists. Much of the data referred to was derived from studies which used positive work exercise, where a significant metabolic demand accompanies the thermal demand. Although there have been a few studies which have used negative work exercise (in which muscles are lengthened in resisting an external load and the metabolic cost is minimal) in an attempt to tease apart the metabolic from the thermal load (6, 10, 15), it remains to be seen whether the control of skin blood flow, for instance, is similar to that during positive work exercise, in which there is a much higher muscle blood flow. Because of high skin conductances during negative work exercise (6), there is the possibility that the low demand for blood flow from the muscles spares cardiac output so that it can be sent to the skin for thermoregulatory purposes. The augmented heat transfer which accompanies this extra skin blood flow may be the factor which keeps internal temperature from increasing to the same degree as it does during positive work exercise at a given level of total heat production. Studies of thermal and circulatory controls during negative work exercise may provide us with some clues about physiological controls and regulations in general.

In Chapter Five certain specific influences which enhance heat dissipation mechanisms at a given level of central thermoregulatory drive were discussed. It was pointed out that both physically fit and heat acclimated individuals maintain a lower internal temperature than controls when

challenged by a heat and exercise test (see also, 11, 16).
This is accomplished by an increased responsiveness of
the sweating mechanism, a lowered internal temperature
threshold for sweating (8) and improvement in the sweating
to skin blood flow ratio that accompanies physical training
(12). It should be reemphasized that some of the circulatory
benefits accompanying heat acclimation probably result from
the progressive increase in plasma expansion with time (14).
Increases in plasma volume undoubtedly contribute to cardiovascular stability by increasing central circulating blood
volume, augmenting stroke volume and allowing heart rate
to fall at a given intensity of exercise. In combination with
the increased evaporation and lowered body temperatures,
most of the circulatory adjustments of heat acclimation can
be explained. What needs to be determined is the precise
role of each of these adjustments in the total acclimation
process, to what extent these differ in different individuals
and the possible role of volume and/or osmoreceptors as well
as the plasma proteins in this process.

The beneficial effects ascribed to the increased abilities
for maintenance of plasma volume with continuous heat and
exercise exposure raise the question of whether increased
capabilities for fluid retention have a beneficial effect upon
heat dissipation mechanisms in general or whether the beneficial effects are merely coincidence.   Factors such as
dehydration or Na^+ loading, which affect the plasma volume,
have been shown to increase the steady state internal temperature during exercise, presumably by decreasing the
effectiveness of the sweating mechanism (2, 13). Ekblom,
et al. (1) observed core temperature increases of 0.3 to
0.4° C when subjects exercised in a mildly dehydrated condition as compared to hydration control values. They attributed the increased internal temperatures to reduced sweating.
Greenleaf and Castle (3) found essentially the same results,
but added data to show that hyperhydrated subjects had
reduced internal temperatures in the steady state of exercise.
These data were in agreement with observations by Senay
(13) that evaporative weight loss was negatively correlated
with serum Na^+ and osmolarity. Nielsen (9) also showed
that increased Na^+ concentration in the blood resulted in a
higher steady state of internal temperature during exercise,
which was the result of a reduction in sweating rate. Thus,

there is suggestive evidence that the gradual, creeping increase of internal body temperature during the so-called
steady state of prolonged exercise is the consequence of a
gradual dehydration and associated reduction of peripheral
circulatory and sweating capabilities. It is clear that a systematic study should be made of the circulatory and sweating
characteristics of exercising individuals under different conditions of hydration and plasma osmolarity. Previous data
are limited in that they do not relate the change in the skin
blood flow to internal temperature relation nor the sweating
rate to internal temperature relation; changes in one or both
of these relations must occur if internal temperature is
modified.

    In a recently completed study, Maron, et al. (4) examined
selected thermoregulatory responses of two runners over the
duration of a competitive marathon race on a relatively cool
(18.6° C) day. Both runners underwent progressive increases
in internal (rectal) temperature over the first 40 min of the
race. Internal temperature levelled off around 39.5° C for
the duration in one runner and underwent a secondary increase from 40.0 to 40.9° C between 85 and 113 min in the
second runner. This runner finished the race with an internal
temperature above 41.6° C, among the highest temperatures
recorded without any clinical signs of heat disorder. The
discrete increments in rectal temperature in the second runner probably reflected transient decreases in sweating rate,
which could have been related to transient bouts of dehydration and/or compensatory adjustments in the circulation (to
maintain central venous pressure), which would reduce core-
to-skin conductance of heat and, perhaps, sweating rate as
well. Studies such as this provide insights that are difficult
to obtain from laboratory studies, where certain factors
associated with running (such as the increase in the convective and evaporative heat transfer coefficients) are normally
absent. However, the many difficulties of making measurements in the field cause this type of study to be somewhat
limited in scope. Although the runners were shown to develop
and maintain quite high temperatures during the race, the
mechanisms by which the temperature and circulatory regulatory systems met the body's demands could not be elucidated.

A study such as the one described above is important in that it illustrates significant inter-subject variability under nearly identical conditions. A recurring theme in the previous chapters was the difficulty in obtaining absolute reproducibility in responses between subjects, from a single subject on different days, or, especially, when attempting to characterize a control system with different techniques. Although any given physiological control system has the same superstructure across individuals, it is well established that the thresholds and gain constants of the system are specific to the individual (7). Further, as was emphasized in Chapter Five, the characteristics of the control system may be flexible with different treatments, at different times of the circadian cycle, or, as noted above, in different conditions of hydration. Further, different modes of investigating the control system may result in different characteristics. For instance, increasing the chest skin temperature by irradiation without changing the average skin temperature results in an exponential (with local temperature) increase in chest sweating rate (5). Increments in sweating rate per degree of chest temperature increase are increasingly greater, when all other factors remain constant. If chest irradiation were the sole method of investigation, one would characterize the control of sweating rate differently from that determined from experiments which use exercise as the method of inducing the thermal load. Similarly, Rowell pointed out in Chapter Four that there are complex interrelations between the cutaneous circulatory dynamics and various other reflexes. This is readily seen from his data describing the effect of posture on skin blood flow control, where there are large differences in skin blood flow at a given set of body temperatures between supine and upright exercise. In Chapter Six it was emphasized that the most important determinant of heat flux during swimming was the thickness of the layer of subcutaneous fat. In Chapter Three Brengelmann noted that recent history could have a large effect on the skin blood flow response. Even formerly-accepted phenomena, such as a certain degree of peripheral vasoconstriction at the onset of exercise, are absent in experienced subjects who are engaging in intermittent exercise. Persumably, the muscle pump, some venoconstriction and perhaps other factors combine to maintain cardiac filling pressure and spare the need for cutaneous vasoconstriction in experienced subjects.

We can conclude that the human is a highly complex system. In different circumstances, different strategies may be employed toward the same end, which is continued performance;   hence, inter- and even intra-individual variability. At different levels of plasma osmolarity, for instance, an individual may have markedly different capacities for sweating at a given set of body temperatures. Without a measure of the state of hydration, the sweating response during exercise can be interpreted as extremely variable instead of tightly controlled, which it is. Variability in responsiveness is even more of a factor in studies of the cutaneous circulation, which subserves two control mechanisms, thermoregulatory and circulatory regulatory. Although we now know a good deal about temperature regulation during exercise, our task is to tease apart factors which interact and cause confusion. When we are able to do this, and are able to represent the control systems as such, we will be able to solve some of the problems with temperature regulation during exercise.

References

1. Ekblom, B., C. J. Greenleaf, J. E. Greenleaf and L. Hermansen. Temperature regulation during exercise dehydration in man. Acta Physiol. Scand. 79: 475-483, 1970,
2. Greenleaf, J. E. Blood electrolytes and exercise in relation to temperature regulation in man. In: The Pharmacology of Thermoregulation, edited by E. Schonbaum and P. Lomax. Basel: Karger, 1973, 72-84.
3. Greenleaf, J. E. and B. L. Castle. Exercise temperature regulation in man during hypohydration and hyperhydration. J. Appl. Physiol. 30: 847-853, 1971.
4. Maron, M. D., J. A. Wagner and S. M. Horvath. Thermoregulatory responses during competitive marathon running. J. Appl. Physiol. In press.

5. Nadel, E. R., R. W. Bullard and J. A. J. Stolwijk. The importance of skin temperature in the regulation of sweating. J. Appl. Physiol. 31: 80-87, 1971.
6. Nadel, E. R., U. Bergh and B. Saltin. Body temperatures during negative work exercise. J. Appl. Physiol. 33: 553-558, 1972.
7. Nadel, E. R., J. W. Mitchell, B. Saltin and J. A. J. Stolwijk. Peripheral modifications to the central drive for sweating. J. Appl. Physiol. 31: 828-833, 1971.
8. Nadel, E. R., K. B. Pandolf, M. F. Roberts and J. A. J. Stolwijk. Mechanisms of thermal acclimation to exercise and heat. J. Appl. Physiol. 37: 515-520, 1974.
9. Nielsen, B. Effect of changes in plasma Na^+ and Ca^{++} ion concentration on body temperature during exercise. Acta Physiol. Scand. 91: 123-129, 1974.
10. Nielsen, B. Regulation of body temperature and heat dissipation at different levels of energy and heat production in man. Acta Physiol. Scand. 68: 215-227, 1966.
11. Piwonka, R. W. and S. Robinson. Acclimatization of highly trained men to work in severe heat. J. Appl. Physiol. 22: 9-12, 1967.
12. Roberts, M. F., C. B. Wenger, J. A. J. Stolwijk and E. R. Nadel. Blood flow and sweating changes with exercise training and heat acclimation. J. Appl. Physiol. In press.
13. Senay, L. C., Jr. Relationship of evaporative rates to Serum Na^+, K^+ and osmolarity in acute heat stress. J. Appl. Physiol. 25: 149-152, 1968.
14. Senay, L. C., Jr., D. Mitchell and C. H. Wyndham. Acclimatization in a hot, humid environment: body fluid adjustments. J. Appl. Physiol. 40: 786-796, 1976.
15. Smiles, K. A. and S. Robinson. Regulation of sweat secretion during positive and negative work. J. Appl. Physiol. 30: 409-412, 1971.
16. Wyndham, C. H. The physiology of exercise under heat stress. Ann. Rev. Physiol. 35: 193-220, 1973.

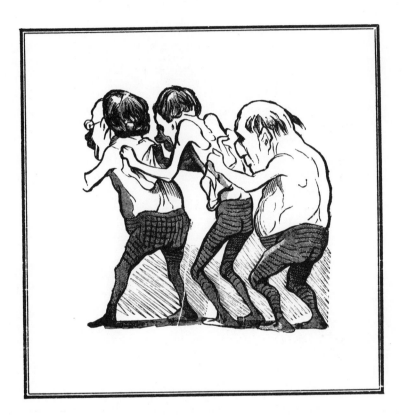

NAME INDEX

A

Aikas, E., 29
Amberson, W. R., 51
Åstrand, P.-O., 18, 19, 102, 103, 104, 105, 106, 108,
    109, 111, 113, 114, 115
Asmussen, E., 50
Atkins, A. R., 32, 104

B

Baker, M. A., 3
Barcroft, H., 37, 50
Barnes, C., 27
Bass, D. E., 78
Beiser, G. D., 71
Benade, A. J. S., 77, 78
Benzinger, T. H., 33, 36, 102, 111
Berg, U., 29, 66, 100, 101, 102, 103, 104, 105, 106,
    108, 109, 110, 111, 113, 114, 115, 121
Bevegård, B. S., 38
Bishop, J. M., 66, 67
Blackmon, J. R., 30, 66, 67
Bleichert, A., 28, 29
Bock, K. D., 50
Braunwald, 71
Breckenridge, J. R., 103, 104
Bredell, G. A. G., 78
Brengelmann, G. L., 27, 30, 36, 37, 38, 39, 40, 42, 45,
    50, 55, 56, 57, 58, 61, 62, 63, 64, 66, 67, 68, 69, 71
Brouha, L., 49
Brown, A. C., 36, 57, 68
Bruce, R. A., 65, 66, 67
Bullard, R. W., 34, 35, 36, 79, 95, 111, 113, 115, 124
Buskirk, E. R., 78

Iriki, M., 2
Irving, L., 113

J

Johnson, F., 113
Johnson, J. M., 36, 37, 38, 39, 40, 41, 42, 45, 55, 56, 57, 58, 60, 66, 67, 69, 71

K

Kang, B. S., 112
Karpovich, P. V., 107
Karvonen, M. J., 29
Keatinge, W. R., 100
Kennedy, J. W., 77, 78, 85, 86
Kidd, B. S. L., 62
Kitchin, A. H., 50
Kitzing, J., 28, 29
Kitzinger, C., 102, 111
Kleeman, C. E., 78
Kraan, J. G., 29
Kraning, K. K., II, 58, 61, 66, 67, 77, 78, 85, 86
Kusumi, F., 30, 64, 66, 67
Kutta, D., 28, 29

L

Lancaster, M. C., 77
Leithead, C. S., 53, 57
Liebermeister, C. von, 5
Lind, A. R., 53, 57
Lofstedt, B. E., 86
Lyons, S. M., 62

M

Magel, J. R., 106, 107
Mager, M., 78
Manalis, R. S., 78
Maron, M. D., 123

SUBJECT INDEX

Acclimation
    beneficial effects, 86, 87, 122
    to exercise, 78, 80
    to heat, 45, 77, 81

Blood flow
    change with acclimation, 84
    forearm, 7, 37, 50, 84
    local temperature effect, 37
    muscle, 13, 37, 50, 51, 58, 66
    renal, 51, 66
    skin blood flow control, 36, 37, 38, 39, 40, 41, 42, 43,
        44, 45, 49, 50, 51, 54, 56, 58, 64, 66, 68, 84
    splanchnic, 51, 66
Blood pressure, 50, 51, 58, 71
    cardiac filling, 54, 62, 71, 87
    venous, 52, 54, 58
Blood volume
    central, 53, 54, 62, 64
    distribution, 39, 50, 51, 57, 62, 64, 68
    muscle, 50
    venous, 50, 52, 53, 54, 55, 57, 58, 62, 64, 87

Cardiac output, 16, 49, 50, 51, 54, 58, 64, 66, 68
Cardiovascular drift, 58, 59
Compliance
    venous, 52, 55, 62
Conductance
    during negative work exercise, 121
    fixed, 94, 96, 97
    minimal, 98, 111, 112, 113
    skin vascular, 56
    whole body, 36, 92, 93, 94, 96, 97, 98, 111, 112, 113,
        114
Control system
    description, 4, 124
    of shivering, 110, 111
    of sweating, 5, 79, 124
    of vasomotor activity, 70, 71, 79
    proportional control, 29, 77, 79